ENDOMETRIOSIS VEGAN DIET COOKBOOK

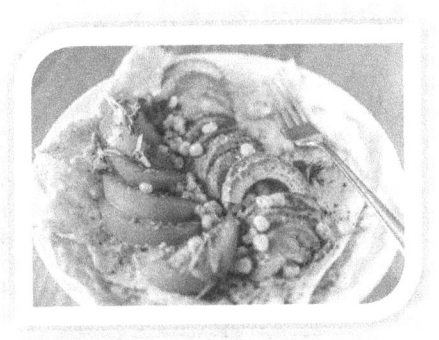

Healthy Plant Based Recipes to Manage Endometriosis

DR. LINDA MCDANIEL

Text Copyright© 2024 by DR. LINDA MCDANIEL

All rights reserved worldwide No part of this publication may be republished in any form or by any means, including photocopying, scanning or otherwise without prior written permission to the copyright holder.

This book contains nonfictional content. The views expressed are those of the author and do not necessarily represent those of the publisher. In addition, the publisher declaims any responsibility for them.

TABLE OF CONTENT

INTRODUCTION — 7

❖ CHAPTER 1 — 9
- ❖ Understanding the Disease, Types, Causes, Symptoms, and Preventive Measures — 9
- ❖ Achieving Optimum Health with an Endometriosis Diet — 14

❖ CHAPTER 2: — 21
- ❖ Benefits of following Endometriosis vegan Diet — 21
- ❖ Complications of Endometriosis if the right diet isn't adopted — 25
- ❖ 14 DAY MEAL PLAN — 29

❖ CHAPTER 3: — 43
- ❖ Endometriosis Vegan Recipes — 43
- ❖ Energizing breakfast: — 43

Berry Chia Pudding — 43
Avocado Toast — 44
Tofu Scramble — 45
Blueberry Oatmeal — 46
Green Smoothie — 47
Coconut Yogurt Parfait — 48
Quinoa Breakfast Bowl — 49
Peanut Butter Banana Toast — 50
Cinnamon Apple Porridge — 51
Vegan Breakfast Burrito — 52
Vegan Breakfast Bowl — 53

Oatmeal with Almond Butter and Berries	54
Chia Seed Pudding with Mango	55
Vegan Breakfast Burrito	56
Sweet Potato Breakfast Hash	57
Coconut Yogurt Parfait	59
Green Smoothie	60
Veggie Breakfast Wrap	61
Chocolate Peanut Butter Smoothie	62
❖ **Tasty Lunch :**	**63**
Quinoa Salad with Roasted Vegetables	63
Lentil Vegetable Soup	64
Mediterranean Chickpea Salad	65
Stuffed Bell Peppers	66
Soba Noodle Stir-Fry	67
Chickpea and Vegetable Stir-Fry	68
Quinoa and Black Bean Salad	69
Vegan Buddha Bowl	70
Vegan Chickpea Wrap	71
Vegan Lentil Soup	72
Quinoa Salad with Roasted Vegetables	73
Lentil Vegetable Soup	74
Mediterranean Chickpea Salad	75
Stuffed Bell Peppers	77
Soba Noodle Stir-Fry	79
Chickpea and Vegetable Stir-Fry	81
Vegan Chickpea Salad Sandwich	83
Vegan Buddha Bowl	85
❖ **Flavorful Dinner :**	**87**
Quinoa Salad with Roasted Vegetables	87
Lentil Vegetable Soup	88
Mediterranean Chickpea Salad	89
Stuffed Bell Peppers	90
Soba Noodle Stir-Fry	91

Chickpea and Vegetable Stir-Fry	92
Quinoa and Black Bean Salad	93
Vegan Buddha Bowl	94
Vegan Chickpea Wrap	95
Vegan Lentil Soup	96
Quinoa Salad with Roasted Vegetables	97
Lentil Vegetable Soup	99
Mediterranean Chickpea Salad	101
Stuffed Bell Peppers	103
Soba Noodle Stir-Fry	105
Chickpea and Vegetable Stir-Fry	107
Vegan Chickpea Salad Sandwich	109
Vegan Buddha Bowl	111

❖ Sweet Snacks: 113

Avocado Toast	113
Mixed Berry Smoothie	114
Hummus and Veggie Sticks	115
Chia Seed Pudding	116
Roasted Chickpeas	117
Sliced Apple with Almond Butter	118
Trail Mix	119
Guacamole with Rice Cakes	120
Edamame Hummus with Veggie Slices	121
Greek Yogurt with Berries and Granola	122
Stuffed Dates	123
Cucumber Hummus Bites	124
Frozen Grapes	125
Rice Cake with Almond Butter and Banana	126
Energy Balls	127

❖ Enjoyable Desserts: 129

Chocolate Avocado Mousse	129
Banana Nice Cream	130
Coconut Chia Seed Pudding	131

Vegan Chocolate Chip Cookies 132
Berry Crisp 134
Banana Nice Cream 135
Coconut Date Balls 136
Baked Apples with Cinnamon 138
Vegan Chocolate Bark 140
Vegan Berry Crisp 142
Vegan Banana Bread 144
Vegan Lemon Bars 147
Vegan Carrot Cake Cupcakes 150
Vegan Chocolate Chip Cookies 153
Vegan Pumpkin Pie 155
Vegan Blueberry Crumble Bars 157
Vegan Chocolate Truffles 159
Vegan Rice Pudding 161

❖ CONCLUSIONS 163

INTRODUCTION

Welcome to the Endometriosis Vegan Diet Cookbook, a comprehensive guide curated with expertise and compassion to support individuals on their journey towards managing Endometriosis through mindful nutrition. As a seasoned nutritionist with years of experience, I understand the profound impact that diet can have on one's well-being, particularly for those navigating the challenges of Endometriosis like tissue outside the uterus, leading to a range of symptoms including pelvic pain, inflammation, and hormonal imbalances. While medical treatments play a crucial role in managing this condition, the power of nutrition should not be underestimated. In this cookbook, you'll discover a wealth of plant-based recipes meticulously crafted to not only provide essential nutrients but also to harness the anti-inflammatory properties of whole foods.

Each recipe is thoughtfully designed to tantalize the taste buds while nurturing the body from within, offering a delicious fusion of flavors and textures that cater to diverse palates.

Through the pages of this cookbook, I aim to empower you with knowledge and inspiration to embrace a vegan lifestyle that supports your journey towards holistic wellness. Whether you're newly diagnosed or have been living with Endometriosis for years, these recipes are tailored to enhance your health and vitality, one nourishing meal at a time.

As we embark on this culinary adventure together, may you find solace, healing, and joy in the transformative power of plant-based nutrition. Here's to reclaiming your health and savoring every delicious moment along the way.

CHAPTER 1

Understanding the Disease

Endometriosis is a complex and often misunderstood gynecological condition that affects millions of individuals worldwide, particularly those of reproductive age. In this comprehensive guide, we will delve into the intricacies of endometriosis, exploring its various types, potential causes, common symptoms, and available preventive measures.

Understanding Endometriosis

Endometriosis is a chronic and often painful disorder characterized by the presence of endometrial-like tissue outside the uterus. This tissue, which typically lines the inside of the uterus and is shed during menstruation, Can implant and grow in other areas of the body, such as the ovaries, fallopian tubes, outer surface of the uterus, and even organs in the pelvis and abdomen. Unlike the normal endometrial tissue, these implants continue to respond to hormonal changes, leading to inflammation, scarring, and adhesions.

Types of Endometriosis

Endometriosis can manifest in various forms, including:

Superficial Endometriosis: Involves small patches of endometrial tissue on the surface of pelvic organs.

Deep Infiltrating Endometriosis (DIE): Involves the infiltration of endometrial tissue into deeper layers of pelvic organs, such as the bowel or bladder.

Endometriomas: Also known as ovarian cysts, these are fluid-filled sacs formed by endometrial tissue within the ovaries.

Causes of Endometriosis:

The exact cause of endometriosis remains elusive, but several theories have been proposed, including:

Retrograde Menstruation: Backflow of menstrual blood through the fallopian tubes into the pelvic cavity, allowing endometrial cells to implant and grow.

Immune System Dysfunction: Abnormal immune response may fail to recognize and eliminate misplaced endometrial tissue.

Hormonal Imbalances: Estrogen dominance or fluctuations in hormone levels can promote the growth of endometrial implants.

Genetic Factors: Endometriosis may run in families, suggesting a genetic predisposition to the condition.

Environmental Factors: Exposure to certain toxins or chemicals may increase the risk of developing endometriosis.

Symptoms of Endometriosis

Endometriosis can present with a wide range of symptoms, which may vary in severity from person to person. Common signs and symptoms include: Chronic pelvic pain, often worsening during menstruation. Painful periods (dysmenorrhea) accompanied by heavy bleeding. Painful intercourse (dyspareunia). Painful bowel movements or urination, especially during menstruation. Infertility or difficulty conceiving. Fatigue, bloating and digestive issues. Adhesions and scar tissue formation, leading to organ dysfunction.

1. **Preventive Measures and Management Strategies:** While there is no definitive cure for endometriosis, several preventive measures and management strategies can help alleviate symptoms and improve quality of life.

Early Diagnosis: Prompt recognition and diagnosis of endometriosis can facilitate timely intervention and management.

Lifestyle Modifications: Adopting a healthy lifestyle, including regular exercise, stress management, and a balanced diet, can help mitigate symptoms.

Hormonal Therapies:

Hormonal contraceptives, such as birth control pills or hormonal IUDs, may help regulate menstrual cycles and reduce pain associated with endometriosis.

Pain Management: Over-the-counter pain relievers or prescription medications may be prescribed to alleviate pelvic pain and discomfort.

Surgical Intervention: In severe cases or when fertility is affected, surgical options such as laparoscopy or laparotomy may be considered to remove endometrial implants and adhesions.

Fertility Preservation: For individuals struggling with infertility due to endometriosis, assisted reproductive technologies (ART) such as in vitro fertilization (IVF) may offer a path to conception.

In conclusion, endometriosis is a multifaceted condition with far-reaching implications for physical, emotional, and reproductive health. By gaining a deeper understanding of its complexities, individuals can empower themselves to seek appropriate medical care, adopt proactive lifestyle changes, and explore various treatment modalities to effectively manage endometriosis and improve overall well-being.

Achieving Optimum Health with an Endometriosis Diet

Nutrition plays a crucial role in managing endometriosis and promoting overall health and well-being.

While there is no one-size-fits-all diet for individuals with endometriosis, making mindful food choices can help alleviate symptoms, reduce inflammation, and support hormonal balance. Here's a guide to the foods to eat and avoid to achieve optimum health with endometriosis:

1. Foods to Eat:

Fruits and Vegetables: Rich in antioxidants, vitamins, and minerals, fruits and vegetables are essential for combating inflammation and supporting immune function. Opt for a colorful variety, including leafy greens, berries, citrus fruits,

and cruciferous vegetables like broccoli and Brussels sprouts.

Whole Grains: Choose whole grains such as quinoa, brown rice, oats, and whole wheat bread, which provide fiber and essential nutrients while stabilizing blood sugar levels.

Plant-Based Proteins:

Incorporate plant-based sources of protein such as legumes (beans, lentils, chickpeas), tofu, tempeh, and edamame to support muscle function and hormone synthesis without the inflammatory effects of animal proteins.

Healthy Fats:

Include sources of healthy fats such as avocados, nuts, seeds, and olive oil, which provide omega-3 fatty acids and support hormonal balance and reduce inflammation.

Herbs and Spices:

Incorporate anti-inflammatory herbs and spices like turmeric, ginger, cinnamon, and garlic into your meals to enhance flavor and promote healing.

2. Foods to Avoid:

Processed Foods: Minimize consumption of processed and refined foods such as sugary snacks, white bread, pastries, and packaged meals, which can exacerbate inflammation and disrupt hormonal balance.

Trans Fats: Avoid foods high in trans fats, including fried foods, margarine, and commercially baked goods, as they can increase inflammation and contribute to hormonal imbalances.

Excessive Dairy: Limit dairy consumption, particularly high-fat and processed dairy products, as they may contain hormones and inflammatory compounds that can worsen endometriosis symptoms. Opt for dairy alternatives like almond milk, coconut yogurt, or soy-based products.

Red Meat: Reduce intake of red meat and processed meats like bacon and sausage, which contain saturated fats and may contribute to inflammation. Instead, focus on lean protein sources such as poultry, fish, and plant-based options.

Caffeine and Alcohol: Limit consumption of caffeine and alcohol, as they can disrupt hormone levels, trigger inflammation, and exacerbate symptoms such as pain and fatigue. Opt for herbal teas and water as hydrating alternatives.

In addition to making informed food choices, it's essential to listen to your body and pay attention to how different foods affect your symptoms. Keeping a food diary can help identify trigger foods and patterns of symptom exacerbation, allowing for personalized dietary modifications.

In conclusion, adopting a nutrient-rich diet focused on whole, plant-based foods while minimizing inflammatory and processed foods can play a significant role in managing endometriosis and promoting optimal health.

By nourishing your body with wholesome foods and avoiding dietary triggers, you can support your body's natural healing processes and improve your overall well-being.

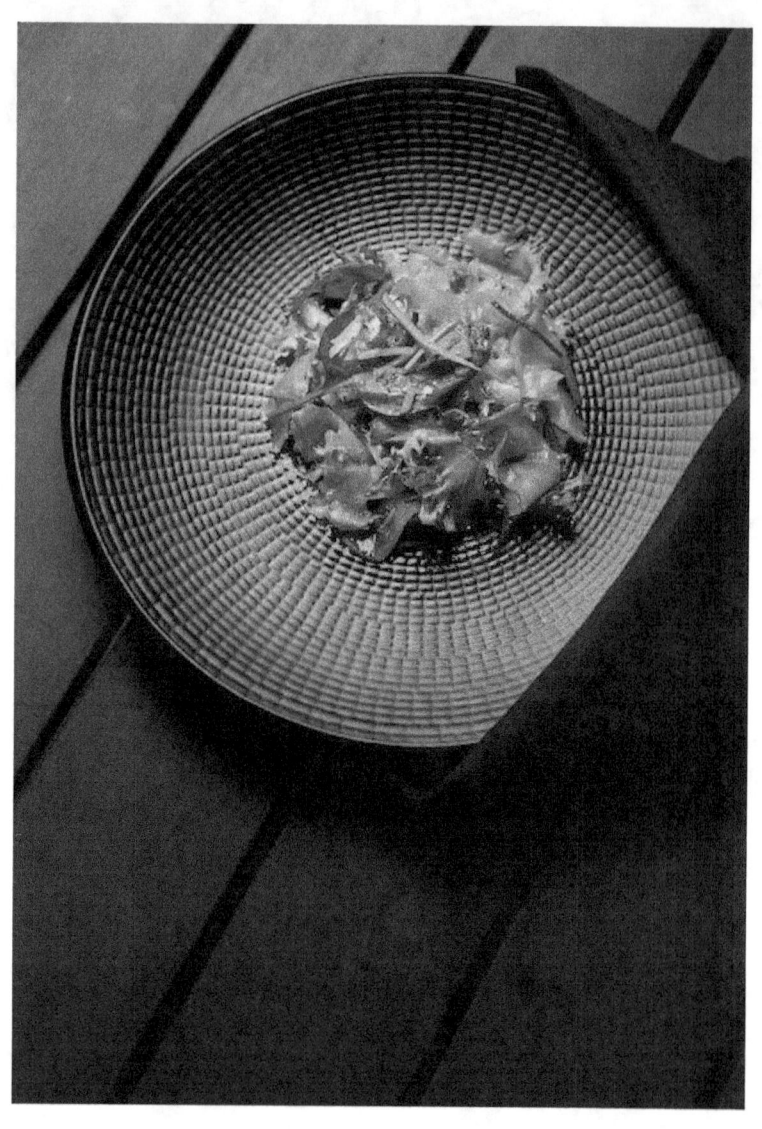

CHAPTER 2:

Benefits of following Endometriosis Vegan Diet

Following an endometriosis disease diet can offer several core benefits for individuals managing this condition:

Reduced Inflammation:

Endometriosis is characterized by chronic inflammation, which can exacerbate symptoms such as pelvic pain and discomfort. By adopting an endometriosis disease diet rich in anti-inflammatory foods such as fruits, vegetables, whole grains, and healthy fats, individuals can help reduce inflammation in the body. Anti-inflammatory foods contain antioxidants and phytonutrients that combat inflammation at the cellular level, potentially alleviating symptoms and improving overall well-being.

Hormonal Balance:

Hormonal imbalances, particularly estrogen dominance, are believed to play a role in the development and progression of endometriosis. Certain foods, such as those high in fiber and plant-based proteins, can help support hormonal balance by aiding in the elimination of excess estrogen from the body and regulating hormone levels. By promoting hormonal equilibrium, an endometriosis disease diet may help reduce symptoms such as menstrual pain, heavy bleeding, and hormonal fluctuations.

Improved Digestive Health:

Many individuals with endometriosis experience digestive issues such as bloating, constipation, or diarrhea, which can further exacerbate discomfort.

An endometriosis disease diet emphasizes whole, fiber-rich foods and minimizes processed and inflammatory foods, promoting digestive health and regularity.

Fiber helps support bowel function, prevent constipation, and promote the growth of beneficial gut bacteria, leading to improved digestive symptoms and overall gastrointestinal well-being.

Enhanced Nutritional Status:

Endometriosis can impact nutrient absorption and utilization due to factors such as inflammation, hormonal imbalances, and digestive dysfunction. Following an endometriosis disease diet ensures adequate intake of essential nutrients such as vitamins, minerals, antioxidants, and omega-3 fatty acids, which are vital for overall health and immune function. By nourishing the body with nutrient-dense foods, individuals can optimize their nutritional status and support their body's natural healing processes.

Weight Management:

Maintaining a healthy weight is important for managing endometriosis symptoms and reducing the risk of complications such as insulin resistance and cardiovascular disease.

An endometriosis disease diet focuses on whole, plant-based foods that are naturally low in calories and high in fiber, promoting satiety and weight management. By adopting a balanced and nutritious diet, individuals can achieve and maintain a healthy weight, which may contribute to improved overall health and well-being.

Following an endometriosis vegan diet offers numerous benefits, including reduced inflammation, hormonal balance, improved digestive health, enhanced nutritional status, and weight management. By making mindful food choices and prioritizing nutrient-rich foods, individuals can support their body's natural healing processes and alleviate symptoms associated with endometriosis, ultimately improving their quality of life.

Complications of Endometriosis if the right diet isn't adopted

If the right diet isn't adopted for endometriosis, individuals may be at risk of experiencing various complications associated with the condition. These complications can significantly impact quality of life and overall health. Some potential complications of endometriosis when the appropriate dietary measures are not taken include:

Increased Inflammation: Endometriosis is characterized by chronic inflammation, and certain dietary choices can exacerbate this inflammation. Consuming processed foods, refined sugars, trans fats, and excessive amounts of red meat can promote inflammation in the body. Persistent inflammation may lead to heightened pain, discomfort, and worsening of endometriosis symptoms over time.

Hormonal Imbalances:

Hormonal imbalances, particularly estrogen dominance, are often implicated in the development and progression of endometriosis. Certain foods, such as those containing hormones or hormone-disrupting chemicals (e.g., pesticides), may contribute to hormonal imbalances. Without appropriate dietary interventions, individuals may experience disruptions in menstrual cycles, increased severity of symptoms, and challenges in managing hormonal fluctuations.

Digestive Issues: Endometriosis can affect the gastrointestinal tract, leading to symptoms such as bloating, abdominal pain, constipation, or diarrhea. Consuming foods that exacerbate digestive issues, such as processed foods, high-fat foods, dairy, and gluten-containing grains, can worsen gastrointestinal symptoms in individuals with endometriosis. Chronic digestive discomfort can significantly impact quality of life and may further exacerbate other endometriosis-related symptoms.

Nutritional Deficiencies: Endometriosis can interfere with nutrient absorption and utilization due to factors such as inflammation, hormonal imbalances, and gastrointestinal dysfunction. Failing to adopt a nutrient-rich diet may result in deficiencies in essential vitamins, minerals, antioxidants, and omega-3 fatty acids. Nutritional deficiencies can weaken the immune system, impair cellular function, and exacerbate symptoms associated with endometriosis, potentially leading to additional health complications.

Increased Risk of Comorbidities:

Endometriosis is associated with an increased risk of certain comorbidities, including infertility, ovarian cysts, pelvic inflammatory disease (PID), and adenomyosis. Poor dietary choices can exacerbate these comorbidities and contribute to their development or progression.

For example, consuming a diet high in inflammatory foods may worsen pelvic inflammation and increase the risk of complications such as PID. Similarly, inadequate nutrient intake may negatively impact fertility and reproductive health.

In conclusion, failing to adopt the right diet for endometriosis can lead to various complications, including increased inflammation, hormonal imbalances, digestive issues, nutritional deficiencies, and heightened risk of comorbidities. It is essential for individuals with endometriosis to prioritize a nutrient-rich, anti-inflammatory diet tailored to their unique needs to mitigate these risks and optimize their overall health and well-being.

14 DAY MEAL PLAN

Day 1:

Breakfast:

Overnight oats made with rolled oats, almond milk, chia seeds, and topped with fresh berries and sliced almonds.

Lunch:

Quinoa salad with mixed greens, roasted vegetables (such as bell peppers, zucchini, and carrots), chickpeas, and a lemon-tahini dressing.

Dinner:

Baked salmon served with steamed broccoli and a quinoa pilaf with diced tomatoes, cucumber, and fresh herbs.

Day 2:

Breakfast:

Whole grain toast topped with avocado slices, cherry tomatoes, and a sprinkle of hemp seeds.

Lunch:

Lentil soup with spinach, carrots, and celery, served with a side of whole grain bread.

Dinner:

Stir-fried tofu with mixed vegetables (such as bell peppers, snap peas, and broccoli) in a ginger-soy sauce, served over brown rice.

Day 3:

Breakfast:

Smoothie made with spinach, banana, frozen berries, almond milk, and a scoop of plant-based protein powder.

Lunch:

Quinoa-stuffed bell peppers with black beans, corn, diced tomatoes, and avocado, baked until tender.

Dinner:

Spaghetti squash noodles tossed with marinara sauce, sautéed mushrooms, spinach, and garlic, served with a side of roasted Brussels sprouts.

Day 4:

Breakfast:

Greek yogurt bowl with mixed berries, granola, and a drizzle of honey.

Lunch:

Kale and chickpea salad with roasted sweet potatoes, pumpkin seeds, and a lemon-tahini dressing.

Dinner:

Baked chicken breast with roasted asparagus and a quinoa tabbouleh salad made with cucumber, tomatoes, parsley, and lemon juice.

Day 5:

Breakfast:

Scrambled tofu with sautéed spinach, cherry tomatoes, and a sprinkle of nutritional yeast, served with whole grain toast.

Lunch:

Lentil and vegetable curry served over brown rice, garnished with fresh cilantro.

Dinner:

Grilled shrimp skewers with roasted vegetables (such as bell peppers, onions, and zucchini) and a side of quinoa pilaf.

Day 6:

Breakfast:

Chia seed pudding made with almond milk, topped with sliced banana, and a sprinkle of cinnamon.

Lunch:

Spinach and arugula salad with roasted beets, walnuts, goat cheese, and a balsamic vinaigrette.

Dinner:

Baked cod fillets with a lemon-herb crust, served with steamed green beans and quinoa.

Day 7:

Breakfast:

Smoothie bowl topped with sliced kiwi, shredded coconut, and a handful of granola.

Lunch:

Mediterranean-inspired wrap with hummus, roasted vegetables, feta cheese, and spinach, wrapped in a whole grain tortilla.

Dinner:

Lentil and vegetable stir-fry with broccoli, bell peppers, carrots, and snap peas, served over brown rice.

Day 8:

Breakfast:

Whole grain pancakes topped with mixed berries and a dollop of Greek yogurt.

Lunch:

Quinoa and black bean salad with diced avocado, cherry tomatoes, corn, and a lime-cilantro dressing.

Dinner:

Baked turkey meatballs served with spaghetti squash noodles and marinara sauce, accompanied by a side salad.

Day 9:

Breakfast:

Avocado toast with sliced radishes, microgreens, and a drizzle of olive oil.

Lunch:

Roasted vegetable and chickpea Buddha bowl with kale, sweet potatoes, tahini dressing, and a sprinkle of hemp seeds.

Dinner:

Grilled tofu skewers with pineapple, bell peppers, and red onion, served with quinoa pilaf and steamed broccoli.

Day 10:

Breakfast:

Smoothie made with spinach, mango, pineapple, coconut milk, and a scoop of protein powder.

Lunch:

Quinoa and lentil soup with diced tomatoes, carrots, celery, and kale, served with whole grain bread.

Dinner:

Baked salmon with a honey-mustard glaze, roasted Brussels sprouts, and a side of wild rice.

Day 11:

Breakfast:

Greek yogurt parfait with layers of granola, mixed berries, and a drizzle of honey.

Lunch:

Spinach and strawberry salad with sliced almonds, feta cheese, and a balsamic vinaigrette.

Dinner:

Vegetable stir-fry with tofu, broccoli, snap peas, bell peppers, and carrots, served over brown rice.

Day 12:

Breakfast:

Chia seed pudding topped with sliced peaches, toasted almonds, and a sprinkle of cinnamon.

Lunch:

Lentil and vegetable curry served over quinoa, garnished with fresh cilantro.

Dinner:

Baked chicken thighs with roasted root vegetables (such as carrots, parsnips, and sweet potatoes) and a side of quinoa pilaf.

Day 13:

Breakfast:

Whole grain toast with almond butter, sliced banana, and a sprinkle of chia seeds.

Lunch:

Mediterranean quinoa salad with cucumber, tomatoes, olives, feta cheese, and a lemon-herb dressing.

Dinner:

Grilled shrimp tacos with avocado, cabbage slaw, and mango salsa, served in whole grain tortillas.

Day 14:

Breakfast:

Smoothie bowl topped with sliced kiwi, coconut flakes, and a handful of granola.

Lunch:

Black bean and vegetable burrito bowl with brown rice, roasted vegetables, salsa, guacamole, and a dollop of Greek yogurt.

Dinner:

Baked cod fillets with a lemon-dill sauce, roasted asparagus, and a side salad.

This meal plan provides a variety of nutrient-rich and satisfying meals to support individuals with endometriosis in managing their symptoms & promoting overall health and well-being. It's important to adjust portion sizes and specific ingredients based on individual preferences and dietary needs.

CHAPTER 3:

Endometriosis Vegan Recipes

Energizing breakfast:

Berry Chia Pudding

Ingredients:

- 2 tablespoons chia seeds
- 1/2 cup almond milk
- 1/4 cup mixed berries
- 1 teaspoon maple syrup

Preparation:

1. Mix chia seeds and almond milk, refrigerate overnight.
2. Top with mixed berries and maple syrup.

Cooking Time: Overnight soaking

Nutritional Value (per serving): Calories: 150, Protein: 4g, Fat: 7g, Carbohydrates: 19g, Fiber: 7g

Avocado Toast

Ingredients:

- 2 slices whole grain bread
- 1 ripe avocado
- Salt and pepper to taste

Preparation:

1. Toast bread and mash avocado.
2. Spread avocado on toast, season with salt and pepper.

Cooking Time: 5 minutes

Nutritional Value (per serving):

Calories: 250

Protein: 6g & Fat: 15g

Carbohydrates: 26g & Fiber: 10g

Tofu Scramble

Ingredients:

- 150g firm tofu & 1/4 cup diced bell peppers
- 1/4 cup diced onions
- 1/2 teaspoon turmeric
- Salt and pepper to taste
- 1 teaspoon olive oil

Preparation:

1. Sauté bell peppers and onions in olive oil.
2. Crumble tofu into the skillet, add turmeric, salt, and pepper.
3. Cook until heated through.

Cooking Time: 10 minutes

Nutritional Value (per serving):

Calories: 180 Protein: 10g, Fat: 10g, Carbohydrates: 8g, Fiber: 3g

Blueberry Oatmeal

Ingredients:

- 1/2 cup rolled oats
- 1 cup almond milk
- 1/4 cup fresh blueberries
- 1 tablespoon maple syrup

Preparation:

1. Cook oats in almond milk until creamy.
2. Stir in fresh blueberries and maple syrup.

Cooking Time: 10 minutes

Nutritional Value (per serving):

Calories: 220

Protein: 6g

Fat: 4g

Carbohydrates: 40g & Fiber: 6g

Green Smoothie

Ingredients:

- 1 cup spinach
- 1/2 banana
- 1/2 cup pineapple chunks
- 1/2 cup coconut water

Preparation:

1. Blend all ingredients until smooth.

Cooking Time: 5 minutes

Nutritional Value (per serving):

Calories: 150

Protein: 3g

Fat: 1g

Carbohydrates: 35g

Fiber: 5g

Coconut Yogurt Parfait

Ingredients:

- 1/2 cup coconut yogurt
- 1/4 cup granola
- 1/4 cup mixed berries
- 1 tablespoon shredded coconut

Preparation:

1. Layer coconut yogurt, granola, and mixed berries in a glass.
2. Top with shredded coconut.

Cooking Time: 5 minutes

Nutritional Value (per serving):

Calories: 280

Protein: 5g

Fat: 10g

Carbohydrates: 40g & Fiber: 6g

Quinoa Breakfast Bowl

Ingredients:

- 1/2 cup cooked quinoa
- 1/2 cup almond milk
- 1/4 cup sliced almonds
- 1 tablespoon maple syrup

Preparation:

1. Mix cooked quinoa with almond milk.
2. Top with sliced almonds and maple syrup.

Cooking Time: 5 minutes

Nutritional Value (per serving):

Calories: 280

Protein: 8g

Fat: 10g

Carbohydrates: 40g & Fiber: 6g

Peanut Butter Banana Toast

Ingredients:

- 2 slices whole grain bread
- 2 tablespoons peanut butter
- 1 banana, sliced

Preparation:

1. Toast bread and spread peanut butter.
2. Top with sliced banana.

Cooking Time: 5 minutes

Nutritional Value (per serving):

Calories: 350

Protein: 10g

Fat: 15g

Carbohydrates: 45g

Fiber: 8g

Cinnamon Apple Porridge

Ingredients:

- 1/2 cup rolled oats
- 1 cup almond milk
- 1/2 apple, diced
- 1/2 teaspoon cinnamon
- 1 tablespoon maple syrup

Preparation:

1. Cook oats in almond milk with diced apple and cinnamon.
2. Sweeten with maple syrup.

Cooking Time: 10 minutes

Nutritional Value (per serving):

Calories: 250 & Protein: 6g

Fat: 4g & Carbohydrates: 45g

Fiber: 7g

Vegan Breakfast Burrito

Ingredients:

- 1 whole wheat tortilla
- 1/4 cup black beans
- 1/4 cup diced tomatoes
- 2 tablespoons diced onions
- 2 tablespoons diced bell peppers
- 1/4 avocado, sliced

Preparation:

1. Fill tortilla with black beans, tomatoes, onions, bell peppers, and avocado.
2. Roll into a burrito.

Cooking Time: 5 minutes

Nutritional Value (per serving):

Calories: 320 & Protein: 10g

Fat: 10g, Carbohydrates: 45g & Fiber: 8g

Vegan Breakfast Bowl

Ingredients:

- 1/2 cup tofu, cubed
- 1/4 cup cooked quinoa
- 1/4 cup black beans
- 1/4 avocado, sliced
- 2 tablespoons salsa

Preparation:

1. Cook tofu in a skillet until golden.
2. Arrange tofu, quinoa, black beans, avocado, and salsa in a bowl.

Cooking Time: 10 minutes

Nutritional Value (per serving):

Calories: 300

Oatmeal with Almond Butter and Berries

Ingredients:

- 1/2 cup rolled oats & 1 cup almond milk
- 1 tablespoon almond butter
- 1/4 cup mixed berries (strawberries, blueberries, raspberries)
- 1 teaspoon maple syrup (optional)

Preparation:

1. In a saucepan, bring almond milk to a boil.
2. Stir in rolled oats and reduce heat to a simmer.
3. Cook for 5-7 minutes, stirring occasionally, until oats are creamy.
4. Transfer oatmeal to a bowl and top with almond butter, mixed berries, and maple syrup if desired.
5. Serve hot.

Cooking Time: 10 minutes

Nutritional Value (per serving): Calories: 320, Protein: 10g, Fat: 12g, Carbohydrates: 45g & Fiber: 8g

Chia Seed Pudding with Mango

Ingredients:

- 1/4 cup chia seeds & 1 cup coconut milk
- 1/2 ripe mango, diced & 1 tablespoon shredded coconut

Preparation:

1. In a bowl, mix chia seeds and coconut milk.
2. Let it sit for 10 minutes, then stir again to prevent clumping.
3. Refrigerate overnight or for at least 4 hours until pudding thickens.
4. Serve chilled, topped with diced mango and shredded coconut.

Cooking Time: Overnight (inactive)

Nutritional Value (per serving):

Calories: 280

Protein: 6g, Fat: 18g, Carbohydrates: 25g & Fiber : 10g

Vegan Breakfast Burrito

Ingredients:

- 2 whole grain tortillas & 1/2 cup black beans, cooked
- 1/4 cup cooked quinoa & 2 tablespoons salsa
- 1/4 avocado, sliced & 2 tablespoons chopped cilantro
- Salt and pepper to taste

Preparation:

1. Warm tortillas in a skillet.
2. Divide black beans, quinoa, salsa, avocado, and cilantro evenly between the tortillas.
3. Season with salt and pepper.
4. Roll up tortillas to form burritos.
5. Serve warm.

Cooking Time: 10 minutes

Nutritional Value (per serving):

Calories: 320, Protein: 10g, Fat: 12g, Carbohydrates: 45g & Fiber: 10g

Sweet Potato Breakfast Hash

Ingredients:

- 1 medium sweet potato, diced
- 1/4 cup diced bell peppers
- 1/4 cup diced onions
- 1 cup spinach
- 1 tablespoon olive oil
- Salt and pepper to taste

Preparation:

1. Heat olive oil in a skillet over medium heat.
2. Add sweet potato, bell peppers, and onions to the skillet.
3. Cook for 8-10 minutes, stirring occasionally, until sweet potatoes are tender.
4. Add spinach and cook until wilted.

5. Season with salt and pepper.
6. Serve hot.

Cooking Time: 15 minutes

Nutritional Value (per serving):

Calories: 280

Protein: 4g

Fat: 7g

Carbohydrates: 50g

Fiber: 8g

Coconut Yogurt Parfait

Ingredients:

- 1/2 cup coconut yogurt
- 1/4 cup granola
- 1/4 cup mixed berries (strawberries, blueberries, raspberries)
- 1 tablespoon shredded coconut

Preparation:

1. In a glass, layer coconut yogurt, granola, and mixed berries.
2. Repeat layering until the glass is filled.
3. Top with shredded coconut.
4. Serve immediately.

Cooking Time: None

Nutritional Value (per serving):

Calories: 250, Protein: 6g, Fat: 10g, Carbohydrates: 35g & Fiber: 7g

Green Smoothie

Ingredients:

- 1 cup spinach & 1/2 cucumber, chopped
- 1/2 green apple, chopped
- 1/2 lemon, juiced
- 1 tablespoon fresh ginger, grated
- 1 cup coconut water & Ice cubes

Preparation:

1. Combine all ingredients in a blender.
2. Blend until smooth.
3. Add ice cubes and blend again until desired consistency is reached.

Cooking Time: None

Nutritional Value (per serving): Calories: 120, Protein: 3g, Fat: 1g, Carbohydrates: 25g & Fiber: 5g

Veggie Breakfast Wrap

Ingredients:

- 1 whole grain tortilla & 1/4 cup scrambled tofu
- 1/4 cup sautéed mixed vegetables (bell peppers, onions, mushrooms)
- 1 tablespoon salsa & Fresh cilantro for garnish

Preparation:

1. Warm tortilla in a skillet.
2. Fill tortilla with scrambled tofu, sautéed vegetables, and salsa.
3. Roll up tortilla to form a wrap.
4. Garnish with fresh cilantro.
5. Serve warm.

Cooking Time: 10 minutes

Nutritional Value (per serving):

Calories: 220, Protein: 8g, Fat: 7g, Carbohydrates: 30g & Fiber: 6g

Chocolate Peanut Butter Smoothie

Ingredients:

- 1 ripe banana
- 1 tablespoon cocoa powder
- 1 tablespoon peanut butter
- 1 cup almond milk
- 1 teaspoon maple syrup (optional)
- Ice cubes

Preparation:

1. Combine all ingredients in a blender.
2. Blend until smooth.
3. Add ice cubes and blend again until desired consistency is reached.

Cooking Time: None

Nutritional Value (per serving):

Calories: 280

Protein: 8g & Fat: 12g

Tasty Lunch:

Quinoa Salad with Roasted Vegetables

Ingredients:

- 1 cup quinoa
- 2 cups mixed vegetables
- 2 tbsp olive oil
- Salt and pepper to taste

Preparation:

1. Cook quinoa according to package instructions.
2. Toss mixed vegetables with olive oil, salt, and pepper.
3. Roast vegetables in the oven at 400°F (200°C) for 20-25 minutes.
4. Mix cooked quinoa with roasted vegetables.

Cooking Time: 30 minutes

Nutritional Value (per serving):

Calories: 320

Protein: 8g

Fat: 12g, Carbohydrates: 45g & Fiber: 8g

Lentil Vegetable Soup

Ingredients:

- 1 cup lentils
- 4 cups vegetable broth
- 2 cups mixed vegetables
- 2 cloves garlic, minced

Preparation:

1. Rinse lentils and drain.
2. Combine lentils, vegetable broth, mixed vegetables, and garlic in a pot.
3. Simmer for 20-25 minutes until lentils are tender.

Cooking Time: 30 minutes

Nutritional Value (per serving):

Calories: 280, Protein: 15g & Fat: 2g, Carbohydrates: 50g & Fiber: 12g

Mediterranean Chickpea Salad

Ingredients:

- 1 can chickpeas
- 1 cup cucumber, diced
- 1 cup cherry tomatoes, halved
- 1/4 cup red onion, thinly sliced

Preparation:

1. Mix together chickpeas, cucumber, tomatoes, and red onion.
2. Dress with olive oil, lemon juice, salt, and pepper.

Cooking Time: None

Nutritional Value (per serving):

Calories: 290 & Protein: 10g

Fat: 14g & Carbohydrates: 35g

Fiber: 10g

Stuffed Bell Peppers

Ingredients:

- 4 large bell peppers & 1 cup cooked quinoa
- 1 cup black beans & 1 cup corn kernels
- 1/2 cup diced tomatoes & 1/4 cup diced onions
- 2 cloves garlic, minced

Preparation:

1. Preheat oven to 375°F (190°C).
2. Cut tops off bell peppers and remove seeds.
3. Mix cooked quinoa, black beans, corn, tomatoes, onions, and garlic.
4. Stuff peppers with the mixture and bake for 30-35 minutes.

Cooking Time: 40 minutes

Nutritional Value (per serving):

Calories: 320 & Protein: 12g

Fat: 3g & Carbohydrates: 60g

Fiber: 12g

Soba Noodle Stir-Fry

Ingredients:

- 8 oz soba noodles
- 2 cups mixed vegetables
- 2 tbsp soy sauce
- 1 tbsp sesame oil

Preparation:

1. Cook soba noodles according to package instructions.
2. Stir-fry mixed vegetables in sesame oil.
3. Add cooked noodles and soy sauce to the pan.

Cooking Time: 20 minutes

Nutritional Value (per serving):

Calories: 340 & Protein: 12g

Fat: 6g & Carbohydrates: 60g

Fiber: 8g

Chickpea and Vegetable Stir-Fry

Ingredients:

- 1 can chickpeas
- 2 cups mixed vegetables
- 2 tbsp soy sauce
- 1 tbsp sesame oil

Preparation:

1. Drain and rinse chickpeas.
2. Stir-fry mixed vegetables and chickpeas in sesame oil.
3. Add soy sauce and cook until vegetables are tender.

Cooking Time: 15 minutes

Nutritional Value (per serving):

Calories: 320, Protein: 10g, Fat: 7g, Carbohydrates: 45g, Fiber: 10g

Quinoa and Black Bean Salad

Ingredients:

- 1 cup cooked quinoa
- 1 can black beans
- 1 cup diced tomatoes
- 1/4 cup chopped cilantro
- 1 avocado, diced

Preparation:

1. Mix together cooked quinoa, black beans, tomatoes, cilantro, and avocado.
2. Dress with lime juice, olive oil, salt, and pepper.

Cooking Time: 20 minutes (includes quinoa cooking time)

Nutritional Value (per serving): Calories: 330, Protein: 12g, Fat: 10g, Carbohydrates: 50g, Fiber: 15g

Vegan Buddha Bowl

Ingredients:

- 1 cup cooked brown rice & 1/2 cup cooked lentils
- 1 cup mixed greens & 1/4 cup shredded carrots
- 1/4 cup sliced cucumber & 2 tbsp tahini dressing

Preparation:

1. Arrange brown rice, lentils, mixed greens, carrots, and cucumber in a bowl.
2. Drizzle with tahini dressing.

Cooking Time: 25 minutes (includes rice and lentil cooking time)

Nutritional Value (per serving): Calories: 320, Protein: 14g, Fat: 10g, Carbohydrates: 45g, Fiber: 10g

Vegan Chickpea Wrap

Ingredients:

- 1 whole grain wrap
- 1/2 cup mashed chickpeas
- 1/4 cup diced tomatoes
- 1/4 cup shredded lettuce
- 2 tbsp hummus

Preparation:

1. Spread hummus on the wrap.
2. Fill with mashed chickpeas, tomatoes, and lettuce.
3. Roll up and slice in half.

Cooking Time: None

Nutritional Value (per serving):

Calories: 280 Protein: 10g, Fat: 8g, Carbohydrates: 40g, Fiber: 10g

Vegan Lentil Soup

Ingredients:

- 1 cup dried lentils & 4 cups vegetable broth
- 1 cup diced potatoes & 1/2 cup diced carrots
- 1/4 cup diced celery & 2 cloves garlic, minced

Preparation:

1. Rinse lentils and drain.
2. Combine lentils, vegetable broth, potatoes, carrots, celery, and garlic in a pot.
3. Simmer for 25-30 minutes until lentils and vegetables are tender.

Cooking Time: 35 minutes

Nutritional Value (per serving):

Calories: 280, Protein: 15g, Fat: 2g, Carbohydrates: 50g, Fiber: 12gickpea

Quinoa Salad with Roasted Vegetables

Ingredients:

- 1 cup quinoa
- 2 cups mixed vegetables (bell peppers, zucchini, cherry tomatoes)
- 2 tablespoons olive oil & 1 tablespoon balsamic vinegar
- Salt and pepper to taste & Fresh herbs for garnish

Preparation:

1. Cook quinoa according to package instructions and let it cool.
2. Toss mixed vegetables with olive oil, balsamic vinegar, salt, and pepper.
3. Roast vegetables in the oven at 400°F (200°C) for 20-25 minutes until tender.
4. Mix quinoa with roasted vegetables and garnish with fresh herbs.
5. Serve warm or chilled.

Cooking Time: 30 minutes

Nutritional Value (per serving): Calories: 320, Protein: 8g, Fat: 12g, Carbohydrates: 45g, Fiber: 8g

Lentil Vegetable Soup

Ingredients:

- 1 cup dried lentils & 4 cups vegetable broth
- 2 cups chopped vegetables (carrots, celery, onions)
- 2 cloves garlic, minced & 1 teaspoon dried thyme
- Salt and pepper to taste & Fresh parsley for garnish

Preparation:

1. Rinse lentils under cold water and drain.
2. In a large pot, combine lentils, vegetable broth, chopped vegetables, garlic, and thyme.
3. Bring to a boil, then simmer for 20-25 minutes until lentils are tender.
4. Season with salt and pepper.
5. Garnish with fresh parsley before serving.

Cooking Time: 30 minutes

Nutritional Value (per serving):

Calories: 280, Protein: 15g, Fat: 2g, Carbohydrates: 50g, Fiber: 12g

Mediterranean Chickpea Salad

Ingredients:

- 1 can chickpeas, drained and rinsed
- 1 cup cucumber, diced
- 1 cup cherry tomatoes, halved
- 1/4 cup red onion, thinly sliced
- 1/4 cup Kalamata olives, pitted
- 2 tablespoons olive oil
- 1 tablespoon lemon juice
- 1 teaspoon dried oregano
- Salt and pepper to taste
- Fresh parsley for garnish

Preparation:

1. Combine chickpeas, cucumber, cherry tomatoes, red onion, and olives in a bowl.

2. In a small bowl, whisk together olive oil, lemon juice, dried oregano, salt, and pepper.

3. Pour dressing over salad and toss to coat.

4. Garnish with fresh parsley.

Cooking Time: None

Nutritional Value (per serving):

Calories: 290

Protein: 10g

Fat: 14g

Carbohydrates: 35g

Fiber: 10g

Stuffed Bell Peppers

Ingredients:

- 4 large bell peppers, halved and seeded
- 1 cup cooked quinoa
- 1 cup black beans, cooked
- 1 cup corn kernels
- 1 cup diced tomatoes
- 1/2 cup diced onions
- 2 cloves garlic, minced
- 1 teaspoon chili powder
- 1/2 teaspoon cumin
- Salt and pepper to taste
- Fresh cilantro for garnish

Preparation:

1. Preheat oven to 375°F (190°C).

2. Place bell pepper halves in a baking dish.

3. Mix quinoa, black beans, corn, tomatoes, onions, garlic, chili powder, cumin, salt, and pepper in a bowl.

4. Spoon mixture into bell pepper halves.

5. Cover with foil and bake for 30-35 minutes until peppers are tender.

6. Garnish with fresh cilantro before serving.

Cooking Time: 45 minutes

Nutritional Value (per serving):

Calories: 320

Protein: 12g

Fat: 3g

Carbohydrates: 60g

Fiber: 12g

Soba Noodle Stir-Fry

Ingredients:

- 8 oz soba noodles
- 2 cups mixed vegetables (broccoli, bell peppers, snap peas)
- 1/4 cup sliced mushrooms
- 2 cloves garlic, minced
- 2 tablespoons soy sauce
- 1 tablespoon sesame oil
- 1 tablespoon rice vinegar
- 1 teaspoon maple syrup
- Sesame seeds for garnish

Preparation:

1. Cook soba noodles according to package instructions.

2. Stir-fry mixed vegetables, mushrooms, and garlic in sesame oil.

3. In a bowl, whisk together soy sauce, rice vinegar, and maple syrup.

4. Add cooked noodles and sauce to the skillet.

5. Cook for 2-3 minutes until heated through.

6. Garnish with sesame seeds.

Cooking Time: 20 minutes

Nutritional Value (per serving):

Calories: 340

Protein: 12g

Fat: 6g

Carbohydrates: 60g

Fiber: 8g

Chickpea and Vegetable Stir-Fry

Ingredients:

- 1 can chickpeas, drained and rinsed
- 2 cups mixed vegetables (bell peppers, broccoli, carrots)
- 1/4 cup diced onions
- 2 cloves garlic, minced
- 2 tablespoons soy sauce
- 1 tablespoon sesame oil
- 1 tablespoon rice vinegar
- 1 teaspoon maple syrup

Preparation:

1. Sauté onions and garlic in sesame oil.
2. Add mixed vegetables and chickpeas.
3. In a bowl, whisk together soy sauce, rice vinegar, and maple syrup.

4. Add sauce to the skillet and cook until vegetables are tender.

5. Serve hot.

Cooking Time: 15 minutes

Nutritional Value (per serving):

Calories: 320

Protein: 10g

Fat: 7g

Carbohydrates: 45g

Fiber: 10g

Vegan Chickpea Salad Sandwich

Ingredients:

- 1 can chickpeas, mashed
- 1/4 cup diced celery
- 2 tablespoons diced red onion
- 2 tablespoons vegan mayonnaise
- 1 tablespoon Dijon mustard
- 1 tablespoon lemon juice
- Salt and pepper to taste
- Lettuce leaves
- Whole grain bread slices

Preparation:

1. In a bowl, mix mashed chickpeas, celery, red onion, vegan mayonnaise, Dijon mustard, lemon juice, salt, and pepper.

2. Spread chickpea salad on bread slices.

3. Add lettuce leaves.

4. Serve as sandwiches.

Cooking Time: 10 minutes

Nutritional Value (per serving):

Calories: 280

Protein: 8g

Fat: 10g

Carbohydrates: 40g

Fiber: 8g

Vegan Buddha Bowl

Ingredients:

- 1 cup cooked quinoa
- 1/2 cup cooked black beans
- 1/2 cup cubed tofu
- 1 cup mixed vegetables (such as kale, carrots, bell peppers)
- 1/4 avocado, sliced
- 2 tablespoons tahini dressing
- 1 tablespoon lemon juice
- Salt and pepper to taste

Preparation:

1. Arrange cooked quinoa, black beans, cubed tofu, and mixed vegetables in a bowl.
2. Drizzle with tahini dressing and lemon juice.

3. Season with salt and pepper.

4. Top with sliced avocado.

5. Serve immediately.

Cooking Time: 20 minutes

Nutritional Value (per serving):

Calories: 350

Protein: 18g

Fat: 15g

Carbohydrates: 45g

Fiber: 12g

Flavorful Dinner:

Quinoa Salad with Roasted Vegetables

Ingredients:

- 1 cup quinoa & 2 cups mixed vegetables
- 2 tbsp olive oil & Salt and pepper to taste

Preparation:

1. Cook quinoa according to package instructions.
2. Toss mixed vegetables with olive oil, salt, and pepper.
3. Roast vegetables in the oven at 400°F (200°C) for 20-25 minutes.
4. Mix cooked quinoa with roasted vegetables.

Cooking Time: 30 minutes

Nutritional Value (per serving): Calories: 320, Protein: 8g, Fat: 12g, Carbohydrates: 45g & Fiber: 8g

Lentil Vegetable Soup

Ingredients:

- 1 cup lentils
- 4 cups vegetable broth
- 2 cups mixed vegetables
- 2 cloves garlic, minced

Preparation:

1. Rinse lentils and drain.
2. Combine lentils, vegetable broth, mixed vegetables, and garlic in a pot.
3. Simmer for 20-25 minutes until lentils are tender.

Cooking Time: 30 minutes

Nutritional Value (per serving):

Calories: 280, Protein: 15g, Fat: 2g, Carbohydrates: 50g & Fiber: 12g

Mediterranean Chickpea Salad

Ingredients:

- 1 can chickpeas
- 1 cup cucumber, diced
- 1 cup cherry tomatoes, halved
- 1/4 cup red onion, thinly sliced

Preparation:

1. Mix together chickpeas, cucumber, tomatoes, and red onion.
2. Dress with olive oil, lemon juice, salt, and pepper.

Cooking Time: None

Nutritional Value (per serving):

Calories: 290

Protein: 10g

Fat: 14g

Carbohydrates: 35g & Fiber: 10g

Stuffed Bell Peppers

Ingredients:

- 4 large bell peppers & 1 cup cooked quinoa
- 1 cup black beans & 1 cup corn kernels
- 1/2 cup diced tomatoes & 1/4 cup diced onions
- 2 cloves garlic, minced

Preparation:

1. Preheat oven to 375°F (190°C).
2. Cut tops off bell peppers and remove seeds.
3. Mix cooked quinoa, black beans, corn, tomatoes, onions, and garlic.
4. Stuff peppers with the mixture and bake for 30-35 minutes.

Cooking Time: 40 minutes

Nutritional Value (per serving):

Calories: 320

Protein: 12g, Fat: 3g, Carbohydrates: 60g & Fiber: 12g

Soba Noodle Stir-Fry

Ingredients:

- ❖ 8 oz soba noodles & 2 cups mixed vegetables
- ❖ 2 tbsp soy sauce & 1 tbsp sesame oil

Preparation:

1. Cook soba noodles according to package instructions.
2. Stir-fry mixed vegetables in sesame oil.
3. Add cooked noodles and soy sauce to the pan.

Cooking Time: 20 minutes

Nutritional Value (per serving):

Calories: 340

Protein: 12g

Fat: 6g

Carbohydrates: 60g & Fiber: 8g

Chickpea and Vegetable Stir-Fry

Ingredients:

- 1 can chickpeas
- 2 cups mixed vegetables
- 2 tbsp soy sauce
- 1 tbsp sesame oil

Preparation:

1. Drain and rinse chickpeas.
2. Stir-fry mixed vegetables and chickpeas in sesame oil.
3. Add soy sauce and cook until vegetables are tender.

Cooking Time: 15 minutes

Nutritional Value (per serving):

Calories: 320 & Protein: 10g

Fat: 7g, Carbohydrates: 45g & Fiber: 10g

Quinoa and Black Bean Salad

Ingredients:

- 1 cup cooked quinoa & 1 can black beans
- 1 cup diced tomatoes & 1/4 cup chopped cilantro
- 1 avocado, diced

Preparation:

1. Mix together cooked quinoa, black beans, tomatoes, cilantro, and avocado.
2. Dress with lime juice, olive oil, salt, and pepper.

Cooking Time: 20 minutes (includes quinoa cooking time)

Nutritional Value (per serving):

Calories: 330 & Protein: 12g

Fat: 10g & Carbohydrates: 50g

Fiber: 15g

Vegan Buddha Bowl

Ingredients:

- 1 cup cooked brown rice & 1/2 cup cooked lentils
- 1 cup mixed greens & 1/4 cup shredded carrots
- 1/4 cup sliced cucumber & 2 tbsp tahini dressing

Preparation:

1. Arrange brown rice, lentils, mixed greens, carrots, and cucumber in a bowl.
2. Drizzle with tahini dressing.

Cooking Time: 25 minutes (includes rice and lentil cooking time)

Nutritional Value (per serving):

Calories: 320 & Protein: 14g

Fat: 10g & Carbohydrates: 45g

Fiber: 10g

Vegan Chickpea Wrap

Ingredients:

- 1 whole grain wrap
- 1/2 cup mashed chickpeas
- 1/4 cup diced tomatoes
- 1/4 cup shredded lettuce
- 2 tbsp hummus

Preparation:

1. Spread hummus on the wrap.
2. Fill with mashed chickpeas, tomatoes, and lettuce.
3. Roll up and slice in half.

Cooking Time: None

Nutritional Value (per serving):

Calories: 280, Protein: 10g, Fat: 8g, Carbohydrates: 40g & Fiber: 10g

Vegan Lentil Soup

Ingredients:

- 1 cup dried lentils & 4 cups vegetable broth
- 1 cup diced potatoes & 1/2 cup diced carrots
- 1/4 cup diced celery & 2 cloves garlic, minced

Preparation:

1. Rinse lentils and drain.
2. Combine lentils, vegetable broth, potatoes, carrots, celery, and garlic in a pot.
3. Simmer for 25-30 minutes until lentils and vegetables are tender.

Cooking Time: 35 minutes

Nutritional Value (per serving):

Calories: 280 & Protein: 15g

Fat: 2g, Carbohydrates: 50g & Fiber: 12g

Quinoa Salad with Roasted Vegetables

Ingredients:

- 1 cup quinoa
- 2 cups mixed vegetables (bell peppers, zucchini, cherry tomatoes)
- 2 tablespoons olive oil
- 1 tablespoon balsamic vinegar
- Salt and pepper to taste
- Fresh herbs for garnish

Preparation:

1. Cook quinoa according to package instructions and let it cool.
2. Toss mixed vegetables with olive oil, balsamic vinegar, salt, and pepper.
3. Roast vegetables in the oven at 400°F (200°C) for 20-25 minutes until tender.

4. Mix quinoa with roasted vegetables and garnish with fresh herbs.

5. Serve warm or chilled.

Cooking Time: 30 minutes

Nutritional Value (per serving):

Calories: 320

Protein: 8g

Fat: 12g

Carbohydrates: 45g

Fiber: 8g

Lentil Vegetable Soup

Ingredients:

- 1 cup dried lentils
- 4 cups vegetable broth
- 2 cups chopped vegetables (carrots, celery, onions)
- 2 cloves garlic, minced
- 1 teaspoon dried thyme
- Salt and pepper to taste
- Fresh parsley for garnish

Preparation:

1. Rinse lentils under cold water and drain.
2. In a large pot, combine lentils, vegetable broth, chopped vegetables, garlic, and thyme.

3. Bring to a boil, then simmer for 20-25 minutes until lentils are tender.

4. Season with salt and pepper.

5. Garnish with fresh parsley before serving.

Cooking Time: 30 minutes

Nutritional Value (per serving):

Calories: 280

Protein: 15g

Fat: 2g

Carbohydrates: 50g

Fiber: 12g

Mediterranean Chickpea Salad

Ingredients:

- 1 can chickpeas, drained and rinsed
- 1 cup cucumber, diced
- 1 cup cherry tomatoes, halved
- 1/4 cup red onion, thinly sliced
- 1/4 cup Kalamata olives, pitted
- 2 tablespoons olive oil
- 1 tablespoon lemon juice
- 1 teaspoon dried oregano
- Salt and pepper to taste
- Fresh parsley for garnish

Preparation:

1. Combine chickpeas, cucumber, cherry tomatoes, red onion, and olives in a bowl.

2. In a small bowl, whisk together olive oil, lemon juice, dried oregano, salt, and pepper.

3. Pour dressing over salad and toss to coat.

4. Garnish with fresh parsley.

Cooking Time: None

Nutritional Value (per serving):

Calories: 290

Protein: 10g

Fat: 14g

Carbohydrates: 35g

Fiber: 10g

Stuffed Bell Peppers

Ingredients:

- 4 large bell peppers, halved and seeded
- 1 cup cooked quinoa
- 1 cup black beans, cooked
- 1 cup corn kernels
- 1 cup diced tomatoes
- 1/2 cup diced onions
- 2 cloves garlic, minced
- 1 teaspoon chili powder
- 1/2 teaspoon cumin
- Salt and pepper to taste
- Fresh cilantro for garnish

Preparation:

1. Preheat oven to 375°F (190°C).

2. Place bell pepper halves in a baking dish.

3. Mix quinoa, black beans, corn, tomatoes, onions, garlic, chili powder, cumin, salt, and pepper in a bowl.

4. Spoon mixture into bell pepper halves.

5. Cover with foil and bake for 30-35 minutes until peppers are tender.

6. Garnish with fresh cilantro before serving.

Cooking Time: 45 minutes

Nutritional Value (per serving):

Calories: 320

Protein: 12g

Fat: 3g

Carbohydrates: 60g

Fiber: 12g

Soba Noodle Stir-Fry

Ingredients:

- 8 oz soba noodles
- 2 cups mixed vegetables (broccoli, bell peppers, snap peas)
- 1/4 cup sliced mushrooms
- 2 cloves garlic, minced
- 2 tablespoons soy sauce
- 1 tablespoon sesame oil
- 1 tablespoon rice vinegar
- 1 teaspoon maple syrup
- Sesame seeds for garnish

Preparation:

1. Cook soba noodles according to package instructions.

2. Stir-fry mixed vegetables, mushrooms, and garlic in sesame oil.

3. In a bowl, whisk together soy sauce, rice vinegar, and maple syrup.

4. Add cooked noodles and sauce to the skillet.

5. Cook for 2-3 minutes until heated through.

6. Garnish with sesame seeds.

Cooking Time: 20 minutes

Nutritional Value (per serving):

Calories: 340

Protein: 12g

Fat: 6g

Carbohydrates: 60g

Fiber: 8g

Chickpea and Vegetable Stir-Fry

Ingredients:

- 1 can chickpeas, drained and rinsed
- 2 cups mixed vegetables (bell peppers, broccoli, carrots)
- 1/4 cup diced onions
- 2 cloves garlic, minced
- 2 tablespoons soy sauce
- 1 tablespoon sesame oil
- 1 tablespoon rice vinegar
- 1 teaspoon maple syrup

Preparation:

1. Sauté onions and garlic in sesame oil.
2. Add mixed vegetables and chickpeas.
3. In a bowl, whisk together soy sauce, rice vinegar, and maple syrup.

4. Add sauce to the skillet and cook until vegetables are tender.

5. Serve hot.

Cooking Time: 15 minutes

Nutritional Value (per serving):

Calories: 320

Protein: 10g

Fat: 7g

Carbohydrates: 45g

Fiber: 10g

Vegan Chickpea Salad Sandwich

Ingredients:

- 1 can chickpeas, mashed
- 1/4 cup diced celery
- 2 tablespoons diced red onion
- 2 tablespoons vegan mayonnaise
- 1 tablespoon Dijon mustard
- 1 tablespoon lemon juice
- Salt and pepper to taste
- Lettuce leaves
- Whole grain bread slices

Preparation:

1. In a bowl, mix mashed chickpeas, celery, red onion, vegan mayonnaise, Dijon mustard, lemon juice, salt, and pepper.

2. Spread chickpea salad on bread slices.

3. Add lettuce leaves.

4. Serve as sandwiches.

Cooking Time: 10 minutes

Nutritional Value (per serving):

Calories: 280

Protein: 8g

Fat: 10g

Carbohydrates: 40g

Fiber: 8g

Vegan Buddha Bowl

Ingredients:

- 1 cup cooked quinoa
- 1/2 cup cooked black beans
- 1/2 cup cubed tofu
- 1 cup mixed vegetables (such as kale, carrots, bell peppers)
- 1/4 avocado, sliced
- 2 tablespoons tahini dressing
- 1 tablespoon lemon juice
- Salt and pepper to taste

Preparation:

1. Arrange cooked quinoa, black beans, cubed tofu, and mixed vegetables in a bowl.//
2. Drizzle with tahini dressing and lemon juice.

3. Season with salt and pepper.

4. Top with sliced avocado.

5. Serve immediately.

Cooking Time: 20 minutes

Nutritional Value (per serving):

Calories: 350

Protein: 18g

Fat: 15g

Carbohydrates: 45g

Fiber: 12g

Enjoy your meals!

Sweet Snacks:

Avocado Toast

Ingredients:

- 2 slices whole grain bread
- 1 ripe avocado
- Salt and pepper to taste
- Optional toppings: cherry tomatoes, red pepper flakes

Preparation:

1. Toast the bread slices until golden brown.
2. Mash the ripe avocado and spread it evenly onto the toast.
3. Sprinkle with salt and pepper.
4. Add optional toppings if desired.
5. Serve immediately.

Cooking Time: 5 minutes

Nutritional Value (per serving): Calories: 200, Protein: 5g, Fat: 10g, Carbohydrates: 25g & Fiber: 8g

Mixed Berry Smoothie

Ingredients:

- 1 cup mixed berries (strawberries, blueberries, raspberries)
- 1 banana, peeled and frozen & 1 cup almond milk
- 1 tablespoon chia seeds
- Optional sweetener: maple syrup or honey

Preparation:

1. Combine mixed berries, frozen banana, almond milk, and chia seeds in a blender.
2. Blend until smooth.
3. Sweeten with maple syrup or honey if desired.
4. Pour into glasses and serve immediately.

Preparation Time: 5 minutes

Nutritional Value (per serving):

Calories: 180, Protein: 5g & Fat: 4g

Carbohydrates: 30g

Fiber: 10g

Hummus and Veggie Sticks

Ingredients:

- 1 cup cooked chickpeas & 2 tablespoons tahini
- 2 tablespoons lemon juice & 1 clove garlic, minced
- Salt and pepper to taste
- Assorted vegetable sticks (carrots, cucumber, bell peppers)

Preparation:

1. In a food processor, combine cooked chickpeas, tahini, lemon juice, garlic, salt, and pepper.
2. Blend until smooth and creamy, adding water if needed to reach desired consistency.
3. Serve hummus with assorted vegetable sticks.

Preparation Time: 10 minutes

Nutritional Value (per serving):

Calories: 150

Protein: 6g

Fat: 8g

Carbohydrates: 15g & Fiber: 6g

Chia Seed Pudding

Ingredients:

- 1/4 cup chia seeds & 1 cup almond milk
- 1 tablespoon maple syrup or honey
- 1/2 teaspoon vanilla extract & Fresh fruit for topping

Preparation:

1. In a bowl, whisk together chia seeds, almond milk, maple syrup or honey, and vanilla extract.
2. Let the mixture sit for 5 minutes, then whisk again to prevent clumps.
3. Cover and refrigerate for at least 2 hours or overnight until thickened.
4. Serve chilled with fresh fruit toppings.

Preparation Time: 5 minutes (plus chilling time)

Nutritional Value (per serving):

Calories: 180

Protein: 5g

Fat: 8g, Carbohydrates: 20g & Fiber: 10g

Roasted Chickpeas

Ingredients:

- 1 can chickpeas, drained and rinsed
- 1 tablespoon olive oil & 1 teaspoon paprika
- 1/2 teaspoon garlic powder & Salt to taste

Preparation:

1. Preheat oven to 400°F (200°C).
2. Pat dry the chickpeas with a paper towel to remove excess moisture.
3. In a bowl, toss chickpeas with olive oil, paprika, garlic powder, and salt until evenly coated.
4. Spread chickpeas in a single layer on a baking sheet.
5. Roast in the preheated oven for 25-30 minutes until crispy, shaking the pan halfway through.
6. Let cool before serving.

Cooking Time: 30 minutes

Nutritional Value (per serving):

Calories: 150 & Protein: 6g

Fat: 6g & Carbohydrates: 20g

Fiber: 6g

Sliced Apple with Almond Butter

Ingredients:

- 1 apple, sliced
- 2 tablespoons almond butter

Preparation:

1. Slice the apple into thin wedges.
2. Spread almond butter on each apple slice.
3. Serve immediately.

Preparation Time: 2 minutes

Nutritional Value (per serving):

Calories: 200

Protein: 4g

Fat: 10g

Carbohydrates: 25g

Fiber: 6g

Trail Mix

Ingredients:

- 1/4 cup almonds & 1/4 cup walnuts
- 1/4 cup dried cranberries
- 1/4 cup pumpkin seeds & 1/4 cup dark chocolate chips

Preparation:

1. Combine all ingredients in a bowl and mix well.
2. Portion into individual servings in small bags or containers.
3. Enjoy as a convenient and nutritious snack on the go.

Preparation Time: 2 minutes

Nutritional Value (per serving):

Calories: 200 & Protein: 5g

Fat: 15g, Carbohydrates: 15g & Fiber: 4g

Guacamole with Rice Cakes

Ingredients:

- ❖ 2 ripe avocados & 1 tomato, diced
- ❖ 1/4 cup diced red onion & 1/4 cup chopped cilantro
- ❖ 1 lime, juiced & Salt and pepper to taste
- ❖ Rice cakes for serving

Preparation:

1. In a bowl, mash the avocados with a fork.
2. Stir in diced tomato, red onion, cilantro, lime juice, salt, and pepper.
3. Serve guacamole with rice cakes for dipping.

Preparation Time: 10 minutes

Nutritional Value (per serving):

Calories: 180 & Protein: 3g

Fat: 10g & Carbohydrates: 20g

Fiber: 8g

Edamame Hummus with Veggie Slices

Ingredients:

- 1 cup shelled edamame & 2 tablespoons tahini
- 2 tablespoons lemon juice & 1 clove garlic, minced
- Salt and pepper to taste
- Assorted vegetable slices for dipping (carrots, cucumbers, bell peppers)

Preparation:

1. Cook edamame according to package instructions, then drain and let cool.
2. In a food processor, combine cooked edamame, tahini, lemon juice, garlic, salt, and pepper.
3. Blend until smooth and creamy.
4. Serve edamame hummus with assorted vegetable slices.

Preparation Time: 10 minutes

Nutritional Value (per serving):

Calories: 150 , Protein: 8g, Fat: 8g

Carbohydrates: 15g & Fiber: 6g

Greek Yogurt with Berries and Granola

Ingredients:

- 1/2 cup dairy-free Greek yogurt
- 1/4 cup mixed berries (strawberries, blueberries, raspberries)
- 2 tablespoons granola & 1 teaspoon honey or maple syrup (optional)

Preparation:

1. Spoon the dairy-free Greek yogurt into a serving bowl.
2. Top with mixed berries and granola.
3. Drizzle with honey or maple syrup if desired.
4. Serve immediately.

Preparation Time: 5 minutes

Nutritional Value (per serving):

Calories: 200 & Protein: 10g

Fat: 5g & Carbohydrates: 25g

Fiber: 5g

Stuffed Dates

Ingredients:

- 8 Medjool dates, pitted
- 2 tablespoons almond butter
- 8 walnut halves

Preparation:

1. Slice each date lengthwise and remove the pit.
2. Fill each date with almond butter and top with a walnut half.
3. Serve immediately.

Preparation Time: 5 minutes

Nutritional Value (per serving):

Calories: 150 & Protein: 3g

Fat: 7g

Carbohydrates: 20g & Fiber: 3g

Cucumber Hummus Bites

Ingredients:

- 1 cucumber
- 1/4 cup hummus
- Fresh parsley for garnish

Preparation:

1. Slice the cucumber into thick rounds.
2. Use a spoon to make a small indentation in each cucumber slice.
3. Fill each indentation with hummus.
4. Garnish with fresh parsley.
5. Serve immediately.

Preparation Time: 5 minutes

Nutritional Value (per serving):

Calories: 50 & Protein: 2g

Fat: 3g & Carbohydrates: 6g

Fiber: 2g

Frozen Grapes

Ingredients:

- 1 cup grapes

Preparation:

1. Wash the grapes and pat them dry.
2. Place the grapes in a single layer on a baking sheet lined with parchment paper.
3. Freeze for 2-3 hours until solid.
4. Serve frozen as a refreshing snack.

Preparation Time: 5 minutes (plus freezing time)

Nutritional Value (per serving):

Calories: 60 & Protein: 1g

Fat: 0g & Carbohydrates: 15g

Fiber: 1g

Rice Cake with Almond Butter and Banana

Ingredients:

- 1 rice cake
- 1 tablespoon almond butter
- 1/2 banana, sliced

Preparation:

1. Spread almond butter evenly on the rice cake.
2. Top with sliced banana.
3. Serve immediately.

Preparation Time: 2 minutes

Nutritional Value (per serving):

Calories: 100 & Protein: 2g

Fat: 5g & Carbohydrates: 15g

Fiber: 2g

Energy Balls

Ingredients:

- 1 cup rolled oats
- 1/2 cup almond butter
- 1/4 cup maple syrup
- 1/4 cup shredded coconut
- 2 tablespoons chia seeds
- 1 teaspoon vanilla extract

Preparation:

1. In a bowl, mix together rolled oats, almond butter, maple syrup, shredded coconut, chia seeds, and vanilla extract until well combined.
2. Roll the mixture into small balls using your hands.
3. Place the energy balls on a baking sheet lined with parchment paper.

4. Refrigerate for 1-2 hours until firm.

5. Serve chilled.

Preparation Time: 10 minutes (plus chilling time)

Nutritional Value (per serving, 2 balls):

Calories: 150

Protein: 4g

Fat: 8g

Carbohydrates: 15g

Fiber: 3g

Enjoyable Desserts:

Chocolate Avocado Mousse

Ingredients:

- ❖ 2 ripe avocados & 1/4 cup cocoa powder
- ❖ 1/4 cup maple syrup or agave nectar & 1 teaspoon vanilla extract
- ❖ Pinch of salt & Optional toppings: sliced strawberries, shaved dark chocolate

Preparation:

1. Scoop the flesh of the avocados into a food processor.
2. Add cocoa powder, maple syrup or agave nectar, vanilla extract, and salt.
3. Blend until smooth and creamy.
4. Divide the mousse into serving dishes and chill in the refrigerator for at least 30 minutes.
5. Garnish with sliced strawberries and shaved dark chocolate before serving.

Cooking Time: 10 minutes

Nutritional Value (per serving)

Calories: 200, Protein: 3g, Fat: 15g, Carbohydrates: 20g & Fiber: 6g

Banana Nice Cream

Ingredients:

- 2 ripe bananas, sliced and frozen & 2 tablespoons almond milk or coconut milk

- 1 tablespoon peanut butter or almond butter (optional) & Optional toppings: sliced bananas, chopped nuts, dark chocolate chips

Preparation:

1. Place frozen banana slices and almond milk or coconut milk in a blender or food processor.

2. Blend until smooth and creamy, scraping down the sides as needed.

3. Add peanut butter or almond butter if desired and blend until well combined.

4. Transfer the nice cream to a bowl and top with sliced bananas, chopped nuts, and dark chocolate chips.

5. Serve immediately.

Cooking Time: 5 minutes

Nutritional Value (per serving):

Calories: 150

Protein: 2g

Fat: 5g, Carbohydrates: 25g & Fiber: 3g

Coconut Chia Seed Pudding

Ingredients:

- 1/4 cup chia seeds & 1 cup coconut milk
- 1 tablespoon maple syrup or agave nectar & 1/2 teaspoon vanilla extract
- Pinch of salt & Fresh berries for topping

Preparation:

1. In a bowl, mix chia seeds, coconut milk, maple syrup or agave nectar, vanilla extract, and salt until well combined.
2. Cover and refrigerate for at least 4 hours or overnight until thickened.
3. Stir the pudding before serving and top with fresh berries.

Cooking Time: 5 minutes (plus chilling time)

Nutritional Value (per serving):

Calories: 200 & Protein: 5g

Fat: 15g & Carbohydrates: 20g

Fiber: 10g

Vegan Chocolate Chip Cookies

Ingredients:

- 1 cup almond flour & 1/4 cup coconut sugar
- 1/4 cup vegan chocolate chips & 2 tablespoons coconut oil, melted
- 1 tablespoon almond milk & 1/2 teaspoon vanilla extract
- 1/4 teaspoon baking soda & Pinch of salt

Preparation:

1. Preheat oven to 350°F (175°C) and line a baking sheet with parchment paper.
2. In a bowl, mix almond flour, coconut sugar, vegan chocolate chips, melted coconut oil, almond milk,

vanilla extract, baking soda, and salt until a dough forms.

3. Roll the dough into tablespoon-sized balls and place them on the prepared baking sheet.

4. Flatten each ball slightly with a fork.

5. Bake for 10-12 minutes until golden brown.

6. Let the cookies cool on the baking sheet for 5 minutes before transferring them to a wire rack to cool completely.

Cooking Time: 12 minutes

Nutritional Value (per serving, 2 cookies):

Calories: 150 & Protein: 3g

Fat: 10g & Carbohydrates: 15g

Fiber: 2g

Berry Crisp

Ingredients:

- 2 cups mixed berries (strawberries, blueberries, raspberries) & 1/4 cup rolled oats
- 2 tablespoons almond flour & 2 tablespoons coconut sugar
- 1 tablespoon coconut oil, melted & 1/2 teaspoon cinnamon
- Pinch of salt

Preparation:

1. Preheat oven to 375°F (190°C) and grease a baking dish.
2. Spread mixed berries evenly in the baking dish.
3. In a bowl, mix rolled oats, almond flour, coconut sugar, melted coconut oil, cinnamon, and salt until crumbly.
4. Sprinkle the oat mixture over the berries.
5. Bake for 20-25 minutes until the topping is golden brown and the berries are bubbling.
6. Let the crisp cool for a few minutes before serving.

Cooking Time: 25 minutes

Nutritional Value (per serving):

Calories: 180

Protein: 3g, Fat: 8g, Carbohydrates: 25g & Fiber: 5g

Banana Nice Cream

Ingredients:

- 2 ripe bananas, sliced and frozen
- 2 tablespoons almond milk (or any plant-based milk)
- Optional toppings: chopped nuts, dark chocolate chips, sliced fruit

Preparation:

1. Place the frozen banana slices and almond milk in a blender or food processor.
2. Blend until smooth and creamy, scraping down the sides as needed.
3. Transfer the nice cream into bowls.
4. Add your favorite toppings, such as chopped nuts or dark chocolate chips.
5. Serve immediately.

Cooking Time: 5 minutes

Nutritional Value (per serving):

Calories: 150

Protein: 2g, Fat: 3g, Carbohydrates: 30g & Fiber: 4g

Coconut Date Balls

Ingredients:

- 1 cup pitted dates
- 1/2 cup shredded coconut
- 1/4 cup almond flour
- 1 tablespoon coconut oil
- 1/2 teaspoon vanilla extract
- Pinch of salt
- Additional shredded coconut for rolling

Preparation:

1. Place dates, shredded coconut, almond flour, coconut oil, vanilla extract, and salt in a food processor.
2. Pulse until the mixture comes together into a sticky dough.
3. Roll the dough into small balls.

4. Roll each ball in additional shredded coconut to coat.

5. Place the coconut date balls in the refrigerator to firm up before serving.

Cooking Time: 10 minutes

Nutritional Value (per serving):

Calories: 120

Protein: 1g

Fat: 5g

Carbohydrates: 20g

Fiber: 3g

Baked Apples with Cinnamon

Ingredients:

- 2 apples, cored
- 1 tablespoon maple syrup
- 1/2 teaspoon cinnamon
- Pinch of nutmeg

Preparation:

1. In a bowl, mix chia seeds, almond milk, maple syrup, and vanilla extract.
2. Let the mixture sit for 5 minutes, then whisk again to prevent clumps.
3. Cover and refrigerate for at least 2 hours or overnight until thickened.
4. In serving glasses or jars, layer the chia pudding with fresh berries and granola.

5. Repeat the layers until the glasses are filled.

6. Serve chilled.

Cooking Time: 5 minutes (plus chilling time)

Nutritional Value (per serving):

Calories: 250

Protein: 6g

Fat: 8g

Carbohydrates: 40g

Fiber: 12g

Vegan Chocolate Bark

Ingredients:

- 1 cup dairy-free chocolate chips
- 1/4 cup chopped nuts (almonds, walnuts, pistachios)
- 1/4 cup dried fruit (cranberries, cherries, apricots)
- Pinch of sea salt

Preparation:

1. Line a baking sheet with parchment paper.

2. In a microwave-safe bowl, melt the dairy-free chocolate chips in 30-second intervals, stirring in between until smooth.

3. Pour the melted chocolate onto the prepared baking sheet and spread it out evenly with a spatula.

4. Sprinkle chopped nuts and dried fruit over the melted chocolate.

5. Sprinkle a pinch of sea salt over the top.

6. Place the baking sheet in the refrigerator for 1-2 hours until the chocolate is set.

7. Once set, break the chocolate bark into pieces.

8. Serve chilled.

Cooking Time: 10 minutes (plus chilling time)

Nutritional Value (per serving):

Calories: 200

Protein: 3g

Fat: 12g

Carbohydrates: 25g & Fiber: 4g

Vegan Berry Crisp

Ingredients:

- 2 cups mixed berries (strawberries, blueberries, raspberries)
- 1 tablespoon maple syrup
- 1/2 cup rolled oats
- 1/4 cup almond flour
- 2 tablespoons coconut oil, melted
- 2 tablespoons maple syrup
- Pinch of cinnamon

Preparation:

1. Preheat the oven to 350°F (175°C).
2. In a mixing bowl, toss mixed berries with 1 tablespoon of maple syrup.
3. In a separate bowl, combine rolled oats, almond flour, melted coconut oil,

2 tablespoons of maple syrup, and a pinch of cinnamon.

4. Spread the berry mixture evenly in a baking dish.

5. Sprinkle the oat mixture over the berries.

6. Bake for 25-30 minutes until the topping is golden brown and the berries are bubbling.

7. Let cool for a few minutes before serving.

8. Serve warm, optionally topped with dairy-free ice cream or coconut whipped cream.

Cooking Time: 30 minutes

Nutritional Value (per serving):

Calories: 250

Protein: 4g

Fat: 10g, Carbohydrates: 35g & Fiber: 7g

Vegan Banana Bread

Ingredients:

- 3 ripe bananas, mashed
- 1/4 cup maple syrup
- 1/4 cup almond milk
- 2 tablespoons coconut oil, melted
- 1 teaspoon vanilla extract
- 1 1/2 cups whole wheat flour
- 1 teaspoon baking powder
- 1/2 teaspoon baking soda
- 1/2 teaspoon cinnamon
- Pinch of salt

Preparation:

1. Preheat the oven to 350°F (175°C). Grease a loaf pan with coconut oil or line with parchment paper.

2. In a large bowl, mix mashed bananas, maple syrup, almond milk, melted coconut oil, and vanilla extract until well combined.

3. In a separate bowl, whisk together whole wheat flour, baking powder, baking soda, cinnamon, and salt.

4. Gradually add the dry ingredients to the wet ingredients, stirring until just combined.

5. Pour the batter into the prepared loaf pan.

6. Bake for 50-60 minutes until a toothpick inserted into the center comes out clean.

7. Let cool in the pan for 10 minutes, then transfer to a wire rack to cool completely.

8. Slice and serve.

Cooking Time: 60 minutes

Nutritional Value (per serving):

Calories: 200

Protein: 3g

Fat: 6g

Carbohydrates: 35g

Fiber: 5g

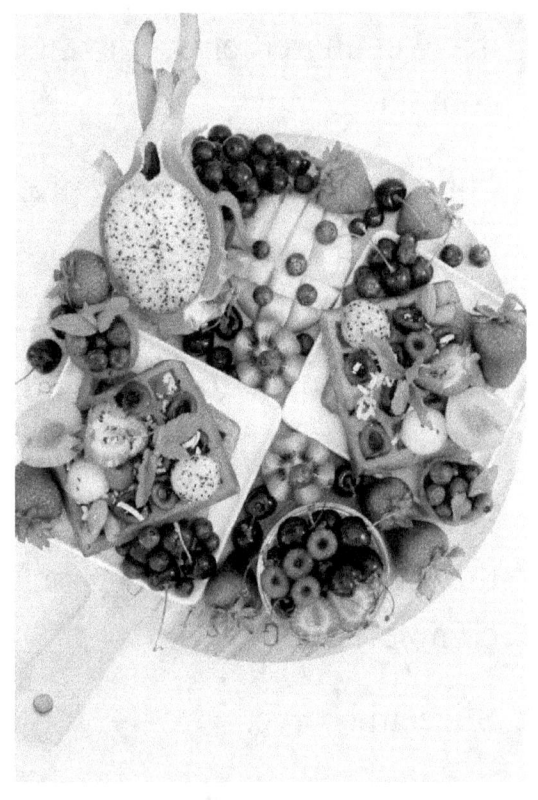

Vegan Lemon Bars

Ingredients:

- 1 1/2 cups almond flour
- 1/4 cup coconut oil, melted
- 1/4 cup maple syrup
- Pinch of salt
- 1 cup raw cashews, soaked in water for 4-6 hours or overnight
- 1/2 cup coconut cream
- 1/4 cup lemon juice
- Zest of 1 lemon
- 1/4 cup maple syrup
- 1 tablespoon arrowroot powder or cornstarch

Preparation:

1. Preheat the oven to 350°F (175°C). Line an 8x8-inch baking pan with parchment paper.

2. In a bowl, mix almond flour, melted coconut oil, maple syrup, and a pinch of salt until crumbly.

3. Press the mixture into the bottom of the prepared baking pan to form a crust.

4. Bake the crust for 10-12 minutes until lightly golden brown. Remove from the oven and let cool.

5. In a blender, combine soaked cashews, coconut cream, lemon juice, lemon zest, maple syrup, and arrowroot powder or cornstarch. Blend until smooth and creamy.

6. Pour the lemon mixture over the cooled crust and spread it out evenly.

7. Return the pan to the oven and bake for an additional 20-25 minutes until the filling is set.

8. Let cool completely, then refrigerate for at least 2 hours to firm up.

9. Slice into bars and serve chilled.

Cooking Time: 40 minutes

Nutritional Value (per serving):

Calories: 220

Protein: 5g

Fat: 15g

Carbohydrates: 20g

Fiber: 2g

Vegan Carrot Cake Cupcakes

Ingredients:

- 1 1/2 cups whole wheat flour
- 1 teaspoon baking powder
- 1/2 teaspoon baking soda
- 1/2 teaspoon cinnamon
- Pinch of nutmeg
- Pinch of salt
- 1/4 cup coconut oil, melted
- 1/2 cup maple syrup
- 1/2 cup almond milk
- 1 teaspoon vanilla extract
- 1 cup shredded carrots
- 1/4 cup chopped walnuts (optional)
- 1/4 cup raisins (optional)

Preparation:

1. Preheat the oven to 350°F (175°C). Line a muffin tin with paper liners.

2. In a large bowl, whisk together whole wheat flour, baking powder, baking soda, cinnamon, nutmeg, and salt.

3. In a separate bowl, mix melted coconut oil, maple syrup and almond milk until well combined. Stir in vanilla extract.
4. Gradually add the wet ingredients to the dry ingredients, stirring until just combined.

5. Fold in shredded carrots, chopped walnuts (if using), and raisins (if using).

6. Spoon the batter into the prepared muffin tin, filling each cup about 2/3 full.

7. Bake for 18-20 minutes until a toothpick inserted into the center comes out clean.

8. Remove from the oven and let cool in the pan for 5 minutes.

9. Transfer the cupcakes to a wire rack to cool completely.

10. Once cooled, frost with vegan cream cheese frosting if desired.

Cooking Time: 20 minutes

Nutritional Value (per serving):

Calories: 180

Protein: 3g

Fat: 8g

Carbohydrates: 25g

Fiber: 3g

Vegan Chocolate Chip Cookies

Ingredients:

- 1 1/2 cups almond flour
- 1/4 cup coconut oil, melted
- 1/4 cup maple syrup
- 1 teaspoon vanilla extract
- Pinch of salt
- 1/2 cup dairy-free chocolate chips

Preparation:

1. Preheat the oven to 350°F (175°C). Line a baking sheet with parchment paper.

2. In a bowl, mix almond flour, melted coconut oil, maple syrup, vanilla extract, and a pinch of salt until well combined.

3. Fold in dairy-free chocolate chips.

4. Scoop tablespoon-sized portions of dough and place them on the prepared baking sheet, leaving space between each cookie.

5. Flatten each cookie slightly with the back of a spoon.

6. Bake for 10-12 minutes until the edges are golden brown.

7. Remove from the oven and let cool on the baking sheet for 5 minutes.

8. Transfer the cookies to a wire rack to cool completely.

Cooking Time: 12 minutes

Nutritional Value (per serving, 2 cookies):

Calories: 150 & Protein: 3g

Fat: 10g, Carbohydrates: 15g & Fiber: 2g

Vegan Pumpkin Pie

Ingredients:

- 1 1/2 cups pumpkin puree
- 1/2 cup coconut milk
- 1/2 cup maple syrup
- 2 tablespoons cornstarch
- 1 teaspoon vanilla extract
- 1 teaspoon cinnamon
- 1/2 teaspoon ground ginger
- 1/4 teaspoon ground nutmeg
- 1/4 teaspoon salt
- 1 prepared vegan pie crust

Preparation:

1. Preheat the oven to 350°F (175°C).
2. In a bowl, whisk together pumpkin puree, coconut milk, maple syrup,

cornstarch, vanilla extract, cinnamon, ginger, nutmeg, and salt until smooth.

3. Pour the pumpkin mixture into the prepared vegan pie crust.
4. Bake for 50-60 minutes until the filling is set and the crust is golden brown.
5. Remove from the oven and let cool completely before serving.

Cooking Time: 60 minutes

Nutritional Value (per serving):

Calories: 200

Protein: 2g

Fat: 8g

Carbohydrates: 30g

Fiber: 3g

Vegan Blueberry Crumble Bars

Ingredients:

- 2 cups rolled oats & 1 cup almond flour
- 1/2 cup coconut oil, melted & 1/4 cup maple syrup
- Pinch of salt & 2 cups fresh or frozen blueberries
- 2 tablespoons maple syrup & 1 tablespoon cornstarch

Preparation:

1. Preheat the oven to 350°F (175°C). Line an 8x8-inch baking pan with parchment paper.

2. In a bowl, mix rolled oats, almond flour, melted coconut oil, maple syrup, and a pinch of salt until crumbly.

3. Press two-thirds of the mixture into the bottom of the prepared baking pan to form a crust.

4. In a separate bowl, toss blueberries with maple syrup and cornstarch until well coated.

5. Spread the blueberry mixture evenly over the crust.

6. Sprinkle the remaining oat mixture over the blueberries to form a crumble topping.

7. Bake for 30-35 minutes until the topping is golden brown and the blueberries are bubbling.

8. Let cool completely before slicing into bars.

Cooking Time: 35 minutes

Nutritional Value (per serving):

Calories: 180

Protein: 3g

Fat: 8g

Carbohydrates: 25g

Fiber: 4g

Vegan Chocolate Truffles

Ingredients:

- 1 cup dairy-free chocolate chips
- 1/2 cup coconut cream
- 1 tablespoon coconut oil
- Cocoa powder, shredded coconut, or chopped nuts for coating

Preparation:

1. In a heatproof bowl, combine dairy-free chocolate chips, coconut cream, and coconut oil.

2. Microwave in 30-second intervals, stirring in between, until the chocolate is melted and smooth.

3. Let the mixture cool slightly, then refrigerate for 1-2 hours until firm.

4. Once firm, scoop tablespoon-sized portions of the chocolate mixture and roll them into balls.

5. Roll each ball in cocoa powder, shredded coconut, or chopped nuts to coat.

6. Place the coated truffles on a baking sheet lined with parchment paper.

7. Refrigerate for another 30 minutes until firm.

8. Serve chilled.

Cooking Time: 2 hours

Nutritional Value (per serving, 2 truffles):

Calories: 150 & Protein: 2g

Fat: 10g & Carbohydrates: 15g

Fiber: 2g

Vegan Rice Pudding

Ingredients:

- 1 cup cooked rice (white or brown)
- 1 1/2 cups coconut milk
- 1/4 cup maple syrup
- 1 teaspoon vanilla extract
- Pinch of cinnamon
- Pinch of salt
- Optional toppings: sliced almonds, dried fruit

Preparation:

1. In a saucepan, combine cooked rice, coconut milk, maple syrup, vanilla extract, cinnamon, and salt.
2. Bring to a simmer over medium heat, then reduce heat to low.

3. Cook, stirring occasionally, for 20-25 minutes until the mixture thickens.

4. Remove from heat and let cool slightly.

5. Serve warm or chilled, topped with sliced almonds or dried fruit if desired.

Cooking Time: 25 minutes

Nutritional Value (per serving):

Calories: 200

Protein: 2g

Fat: 8g

Carbohydrates: 30g

Fiber: 1g

CONCLUSIONS

In conclusion, this Endometriosis Vegan Diet Cookbook offers a comprehensive array of delicious and nutrient-rich recipes tailored specifically to support individuals managing endometriosis. Endometriosis is a complex condition that can significantly impact daily life, and dietary choices play a crucial role in managing symptoms and promoting overall well-being. By focusing on plant-based, anti-inflammatory ingredients, these recipes are designed to help alleviate discomfort, reduce inflammation, and support hormonal balance. Throughout this cookbook, we've provided a diverse selection of breakfasts, lunches, dinners, snacks, and desserts, ensuring that every meal is both nourishing and satisfying. From comforting soups to vibrant salads, hearty mains to indulgent treats, there's something for every craving and occasion.

Each recipe is carefully crafted with ingredients known for their anti-inflammatory properties, such as fruits, vegetables, whole grains, legumes, nuts, and seeds. By incorporating these foods into your diet, you can support your body's natural healing processes and enhance overall health.

As you embark on your journey with the Endometriosis Vegan Diet, remember that small changes can make a big difference. Whether you're transitioning to a fully plant-based lifestyle or simply incorporating more plant-based meals into your routine, every step counts towards improving your well-being. It's important to listen to your body, experiment with different recipes, and find what works best for you.

By nourishing your body with wholesome, plant-based foods, you're not only supporting your physical health but also making a positive impact on the planet.

Plant-based diets have been shown to reduce the risk of chronic diseases, protect the environment, and promote ethical and sustainable food choices.

So, let this cookbook be your guide to delicious and nutritious meals that support your journey towards managing endometriosis and embracing a vibrant, plant-powered lifestyle. Together, let's nourish our bodies, nurture our health, and thrive with compassion and vitality. You deserve to feel your best, and with the power of plants, you can achieve optimal health and well-being.

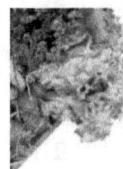

WEEKLY MEAL PLANNER

MONDAY	BREAKFAST		GROCERY LIST	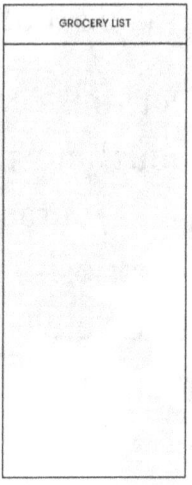
	LUNCH			
	DINNER			
TUESDAY	BREAKFAST			
	LUNCH			
	DINNER			
WEDNESDAY	BREAKFAST			
	LUNCH			
	DINNER			
THURSDAY	BREAKFAST			
	LUNCH			
	DINNER			
FRIDAY	BREAKFAST		SNACKS	
	LUNCH			
	DINNER			
SATURDAY	BREAKFAST			
	LUNCH			
	DINNER			
SUNDAY	BREAKFAST			
	LUNCH			
	DINNER			

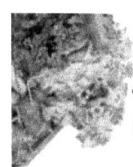

WEEKLY MEAL PLANNER

MONDAY	BREAKFAST	
	LUNCH	
	DINNER	
TUESDAY	BREAKFAST	
	LUNCH	
	DINNER	
WEDNESDAY	BREAKFAST	
	LUNCH	
	DINNER	
THURSDAY	BREAKFAST	
	LUNCH	
	DINNER	
FRIDAY	BREAKFAST	
	LUNCH	
	DINNER	
SARTURDAY	BREAKFAST	
	LUNCH	
	DINNER	
SUNDAY	BREAKFAST	
	LUNCH	
	DINNER	

GROCERY LIST

SNACKS

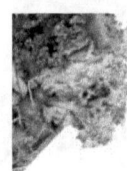

WEEKLY MEAL PLANNER

MONDAY	BREAKFAST	
	LUNCH	
	DINNER	
TUESDAY	BREAKFAST	
	LUNCH	
	DINNER	
WEDNESDAY	BREAKFAST	
	LUNCH	
	DINNER	
THURSDAY	BREAKFAST	
	LUNCH	
	DINNER	
FRIDAY	BREAKFAST	
	LUNCH	
	DINNER	
SATURDAY	BREAKFAST	
	LUNCH	
	DINNER	
SUNDAY	BREAKFAST	
	LUNCH	
	DINNER	

GROCERY LIST

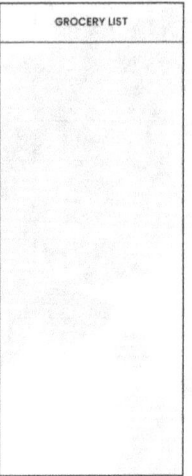

SNACKS

WEEKLY MEAL PLANNER

MONDAY	BREAKFAST	
	LUNCH	
	DINNER	
TUESDAY	BREAKFAST	
	LUNCH	
	DINNER	
WEDNESDAY	BREAKFAST	
	LUNCH	
	DINNER	
THURSDAY	BREAKFAST	
	LUNCH	
	DINNER	
FRIDAY	BREAKFAST	
	LUNCH	
	DINNER	
SARTURDAY	BREAKFAST	
	LUNCH	
	DINNER	
SUNDAY	BREAKFAST	
	LUNCH	
	DINNER	

GROCERY LIST

SNACKS

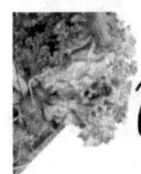

WEEKLY MEAL PLANNER

MONDAY	BREAKFAST	
	LUNCH	
	DINNER	
TUESDAY	BREAKFAST	
	LUNCH	
	DINNER	
WEDNESDAY	BREAKFAST	
	LUNCH	
	DINNER	
THURSDAY	BREAKFAST	
	LUNCH	
	DINNER	
FRIDAY	BREAKFAST	
	LUNCH	
	DINNER	
SARTURDAY	BREAKFAST	
	LUNCH	
	DINNER	
SUNDAY	BREAKFAST	
	LUNCH	
	DINNER	

GROCERY LIST

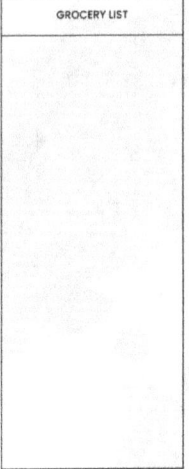

SNACKS

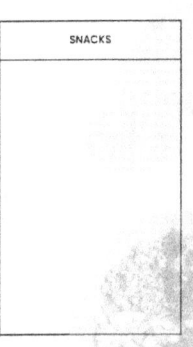

WEEKLY MEAL PLANNER

MONDAY	BREAKFAST	
	LUNCH	
	DINNER	
TUESDAY	BREAKFAST	
	LUNCH	
	DINNER	
WEDNESDAY	BREAKFAST	
	LUNCH	
	DINNER	
THURSDAY	BREAKFAST	
	LUNCH	
	DINNER	
FRIDAY	BREAKFAST	
	LUNCH	
	DINNER	
SARTURDAY	BREAKFAST	
	LUNCH	
	DINNER	
SUNDAY	BREAKFAST	
	LUNCH	
	DINNER	

GROCERY LIST

SNACKS

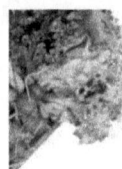

WEEKLY MEAL PLANNER

				GROCERY LIST
MONDAY	BREAKFAST			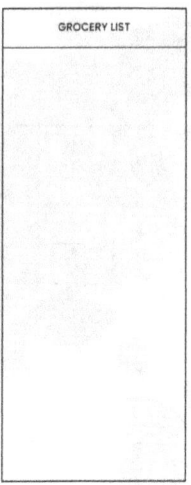
	LUNCH			
	DINNER			
TUESDAY	BREAKFAST			
	LUNCH			
	DINNER			
WEDNESDAY	BREAKFAST			
	LUNCH			
	DINNER			
THURSDAY	BREAKFAST			
	LUNCH			
	DINNER			SNACKS
FRIDAY	BREAKFAST			
	LUNCH			
	DINNER			
SARTURDAY	BREAKFAST			
	LUNCH			
	DINNER			
SUNDAY	BREAKFAST			
	LUNCH			
	DINNER			

WEEKLY MEAL PLANNER

MONDAY	BREAKFAST	
	LUNCH	
	DINNER	
TUESDAY	BREAKFAST	
	LUNCH	
	DINNER	
WEDNESDAY	BREAKFAST	
	LUNCH	
	DINNER	
THURSDAY	BREAKFAST	
	LUNCH	
	DINNER	
FRIDAY	BREAKFAST	
	LUNCH	
	DINNER	
SARTURDAY	BREAKFAST	
	LUNCH	
	DINNER	
SUNDAY	BREAKFAST	
	LUNCH	
	DINNER	

GROCERY LIST

SNACKS

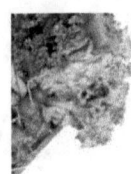

WEEKLY MEAL PLANNER

MONDAY	BREAKFAST	
	LUNCH	
	DINNER	
TUESDAY	BREAKFAST	
	LUNCH	
	DINNER	
WEDNESDAY	BREAKFAST	
	LUNCH	
	DINNER	
THURSDAY	BREAKFAST	
	LUNCH	
	DINNER	
FRIDAY	BREAKFAST	
	LUNCH	
	DINNER	
SARTURDAY	BREAKFAST	
	LUNCH	
	DINNER	
SUNDAY	BREAKFAST	
	LUNCH	
	DINNER	

GROCERY LIST

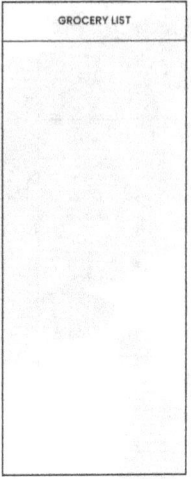

SNACKS

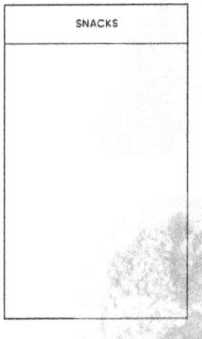

WEEKLY MEAL PLANNER

MONDAY	BREAKFAST	
	LUNCH	
	DINNER	
TUESDAY	BREAKFAST	
	LUNCH	
	DINNER	
WEDNESDAY	BREAKFAST	
	LUNCH	
	DINNER	
THURSDAY	BREAKFAST	
	LUNCH	
	DINNER	
FRIDAY	BREAKFAST	
	LUNCH	
	DINNER	
SARTURDAY	BREAKFAST	
	LUNCH	
	DINNER	
SUNDAY	BREAKFAST	
	LUNCH	
	DINNER	

GROCERY LIST

SNACKS

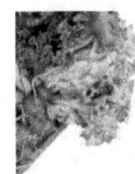

WEEKLY MEAL PLANNER

MONDAY	BREAKFAST		
	LUNCH		
	DINNER		
TUESDAY	BREAKFAST		
	LUNCH		
	DINNER		
WEDNESDAY	BREAKFAST		
	LUNCH		
	DINNER		
THURSDAY	BREAKFAST		
	LUNCH		
	DINNER		
FRIDAY	BREAKFAST		
	LUNCH		
	DINNER		
SARTURDAY	BREAKFAST		
	LUNCH		
	DINNER		
SUNDAY	BREAKFAST		
	LUNCH		
	DINNER		

GROCERY LIST

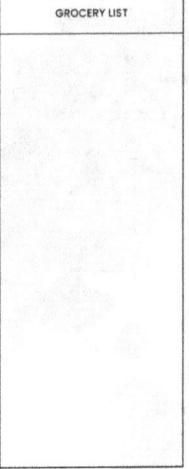

SNACKS

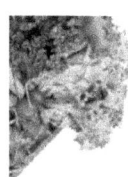

WEEKLY MEAL PLANNER

MONDAY	BREAKFAST	
	LUNCH	
	DINNER	
TUESDAY	BREAKFAST	
	LUNCH	
	DINNER	
WEDNESDAY	BREAKFAST	
	LUNCH	
	DINNER	
THURSDAY	BREAKFAST	
	LUNCH	
	DINNER	
FRIDAY	BREAKFAST	
	LUNCH	
	DINNER	
SARTURDAY	BREAKFAST	
	LUNCH	
	DINNER	
SUNDAY	BREAKFAST	
	LUNCH	
	DINNER	

GROCERY LIST

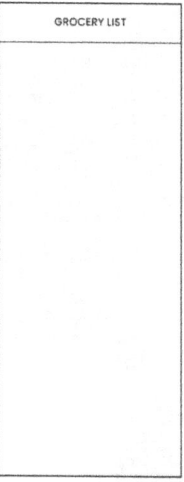

SNACKS

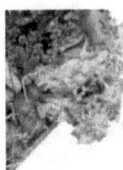

WEEKLY MEAL PLANNER

MONDAY	BREAKFAST	
	LUNCH	
	DINNER	
TUESDAY	BREAKFAST	
	LUNCH	
	DINNER	
WEDNESDAY	BREAKFAST	
	LUNCH	
	DINNER	
THURSDAY	BREAKFAST	
	LUNCH	
	DINNER	
FRIDAY	BREAKFAST	
	LUNCH	
	DINNER	
SARTURDAY	BREAKFAST	
	LUNCH	
	DINNER	
SUNDAY	BREAKFAST	
	LUNCH	
	DINNER	

GROCERY LIST

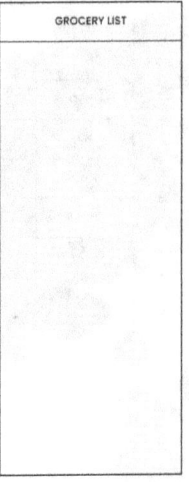

SNACKS

WEEKLY MEAL PLANNER

MONDAY	BREAKFAST	
	LUNCH	
	DINNER	
TUESDAY	BREAKFAST	
	LUNCH	
	DINNER	
WEDNESDAY	BREAKFAST	
	LUNCH	
	DINNER	
THURSDAY	BREAKFAST	
	LUNCH	
	DINNER	
FRIDAY	BREAKFAST	
	LUNCH	
	DINNER	
SARTURDAY	BREAKFAST	
	LUNCH	
	DINNER	
SUNDAY	BREAKFAST	
	LUNCH	
	DINNER	

GROCERY LIST

SNACKS

www.ingramcontent.com/pod-product-compliance
Lightning Source LLC
Chambersburg PA
CBHW050058230526
45470CB00004B/1586